# Recent Advances in

## Paediatrics 29

# Recent Advances in

# Paediatrics 29

**Gautam Kulkarni** MD DNB FRCPCH Dip Allergy

Consultant in Paediatrics and Adolescent Health
The Portland Hospital and Circle Health
Health Tech Adviser
London, UK

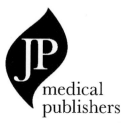

JP
medical
publishers

London • New Delhi

© 2023 JP Medical Ltd.
Published by JP Medical Ltd,
83 Victoria Street, London, SW1H 0HW, UK
Tel: +44 (0)20 3170 8910
Fax: +44 (0)20 3008 6180
Email: info@jpmedpub.com
Web: www.jpmedpub.com

The rights of Gautam Kulkarni to be identified as the editor of this work have been asserted by him in accordance with the Copyright, Designs and Patents Act 1988.

All brand names and product names used in this book are trade names, service marks, trademarks or registered trademarks of their respective owners. The publisher is not associated with any product or vendor mentioned in this book.

Medical knowledge and practice change constantly. This book is designed to provide accurate, authoritative information about the subject matter in question. However readers are advised to check the most current information available on procedures included and check information from the manufacturer of each product to be administered, to verify the recommended dose, formula, method and duration of administration, adverse effects and contraindications. It is the responsibility of the practitioner to take all appropriate safety precautions. Neither the publisher nor the editor assume any liability for any injury and/or damage to persons or property arising from or related to use of material in this book.

This book is sold on the understanding that the publisher is not engaged in providing professional medical services. If such advice or services are required, the services of a competent medical professional should be sought.

Every effort has been made where necessary to contact holders of copyright to obtain permission to reproduce copyright material. If any have been inadvertently overlooked, the publisher will be pleased to make the necessary arrangements at the first opportunity.

ISBN: 978-1-78779-177-0

**British Library Cataloguing in Publication Data**
A catalogue record for this book is available from the British Library

**Library of Congress Cataloging in Publication Data**
A catalog record for this book is available from the Library of Congress

Manager Publishing:      Saima Rashid

Editorial Assistant:      Keshav Kumar

Cover Design:      Seema Dogra

# Preface

I am absolutely delighted to present 'Recent Advances in Paediatrics 29'. With a truly international selection of contributors, this book reflects changes in the age groups of children we look after with an emphasis on adolescent health, both physical and mental. It highlights topical issues such as gender dysphoria, social media use and health challenges specific to adolescents. The chapter on technology in adolescent mental health appraises the current technology and gamification strategies for engaging children with mental health issues.

Advances in perinatal genetics, are presented alongside evidence based updates in neonatology, with an emphasis on stabilisation, respiratory management, family integrated care and advances in screening.

The approach to orthopaedic interventions in cerebral palsy is an exceptionally valuable resource for paediatricians alongside the chapter raising awareness in bone health and osteoporosis.

As paediatricians, it is vital we are closely involved in the care of children undergoing surgery. The chapter on surgical advances highlights the improvements in paediatric surgical outcomes as a result of better medical care pre- and post-surgery. Many conditions, as exemplified by the chapter on posterior urethral valves continue to need long term medical and surgical follow up. There is a strong emphasis on improving the safety of the children we look after by introducing safety check lists and having clear pathways of escalation for sick children.

I am pleased to introduce data and technology in paediatrics, a passion of mine shape the future of healthcare. Striving to do our best for the children we look after, makes us natural innovators and I have no doubt that all paediatricians, both experienced and recently qualified will find this chapter interesting.

As a paediatrician working in London, which is among the most ethnically diverse cities, I am hopeful this book and its chapters will be relevant and inspiring to healthcare professionals working with children and adolescents all over the world.

**Gautam Kulkarni**

# Contents

# Acknowledgements

My personal thanks to my fantastic team at JP Medical Publishers and to all my contributors for their passion in improving healthcare outcomes for children and adolescents.

# Chapter 1

# Adolescent health

*Mathavi G Sankar, Anisha Abraham*

## ADOLESCENCE

The World Health Organization (WHO) defines adolescence as the transition period of life between childhood and adulthood, from ages 10 to 19. It is a critical stage of human development, filled with rapid and unique biological, cognitive, psychological and social changes. Despite being considered a generally healthy period of life, distinctive health and social challenges arise during adolescence, continuing well into adulthood. For example, half of all cases of lifetime mental illness arises before the age of 14 years [1]. Significant preventable and treatable injury and death also occur in the adolescent years. Furthermore, in adolescence, people establish habits and behaviours – related to diet, physical activity, sex, and substance abuse – that directly impact their health now and in the future. Thus, health-care providers must partner with families, educational institutions, community organisations, and governments to address the unique needs of adolescents and ensure their healthy transition into adulthood.

## UNIQUE DEVELOPMENT IN ADOLESCENTS

### Brain development

The hallmark of psychosocial development in adolescence is a gradually gaining autonomy and making individual decisions. Decision-making relies on two systems within the brain: a socio-emotional system and a cognitive-control system. The socio-emotional system, comprised largely of limbic and paralimbic structures, is responsible for a fast, intuitive decision-making that is influenced by reward feelings and autonomic responses. On the other hand, the cognitive-control system, comprised of prefrontal and parietal cortical structures, is a deliberate decision-making process that requires more time and conscious effort. The development and co-ordination of these two systems are not yet fully developed in the adolescent brain. While the socio-emotional system matures around puberty, the

**Mathavi G Sankar** MD MPH, George Washington University School of Medicine and Health Sciences, 2300 I Street NW, Washington, USA.
Email: msankar@gwu.edu (for correspondence).

**Anisha Abraham** MD MPH, Division of Adolescent and Young Adult Medicine, Children's National Hospital, 111 Michigan Avenue NW, Washington, USA.
Email: aabraham2@childrensnational.org (for correspondence).

cognitive-control system does not fully develop until the mid-20s. Integration of these two systems also does not occur until the 20s. Consequently, there is an imbalance between these two systems during adolescence. Since the accelerator (socio-emotional system) overpowers the brakes (cognitive-control system), adolescents are more likely to engage in risky behaviour [2]. On a positive note, adolescents' growing brains allow them to discover new passions and acquire skills such as learning a new language quickly. Thus, it is important for adults to understand how the adolescent brain works to properly guide them and promote good health.

## Physical development

Puberty is the process of physiologic development during which an adolescent reach sexual maturity. Puberty usually starts between ages 8 and 13 years in females and ages 9 and 14 years in boys. During this time, pulsatile secretion of gonadotropin-releasing hormone (GnRH) from the hypothalamus triggers downstream hormone release. As a result, sex hormone (testosterone and oestrogen) levels surge resulting in physical changes, including an increase height and weight, a change in fat and muscle distribution, and body hair growth. The hormones can also affect the adolescent's developing brain, resulting in cognitive and emotional changes [3]. Regardless of where in this world a teen grows up, the overall sequence of physical changes in puberty is the same.

## Pubertal changes in girls

In most girls, the first noticeable sign of puberty is breast bud development (thelarche). Breast buds may initially develop on only one side first, appearing as a hard, tender knot under the nipple. Parents may often bring their child into the paediatrician's office with concerns for a unilateral, tender breast mass. However, in a few months, the tenderness will improve, and breast sizes will even out. In about 15% of girls, hair growth in the pubic region (pubarche) may be the first sign of puberty [4]. Typically, menstruation begins (menarche) in about 2 years after breast bud development [5]. Adolescent girls usually have a growth spurt in this time before menstrual cycles begin (**Figure 1.1**) [6].

While the sequence of puberty is similar in most girls, the timing of puberty onset varies widely among individuals, though some studies show an association with genetics, body mass index (BMI), and race/ethnicity. For example, a longitudinal cohort study of girls in the United States found that median age of breast bud development was 8.8 years in Black girls, 9.3 years in Hispanic girls, and 9.7 years in Asian and White non-Hispanic girls. The study found that BMI accounted for about 14% of the variance, while race/ethnicity accounted for only 4% [7].

## Pubertal changes in boys

In boys, the first sign of puberty on physical examination is testicular enlargement. Boys and parents are often unaware of the early signs of puberty compared to girls, who have more noticeable pubertal changes. In addition to testicular enlargement, the next change in boys is the appearance of pubic hair, which will start out soft and later become curlier and coarse, extending from the pubic area to the thighs. Penile length will also increase, and boys will experience a growth spurt. Afterwards, sperm production begins (spermarche), and sperm can be found in the urine. Boys may experience nocturnal emissions, which can be embarrassing for many teenage boys, who should be reassured that it is a normal part of development.

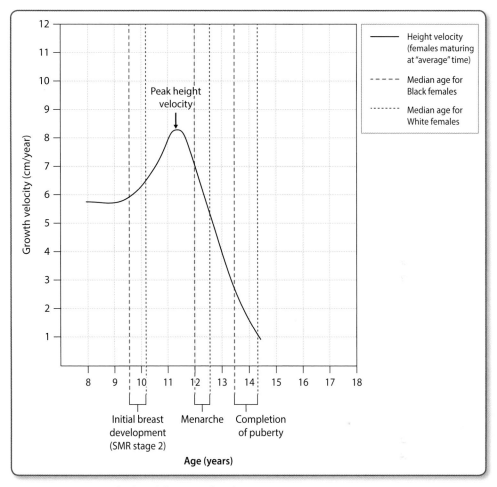

**Figure 1.1** Sequence of pubertal changes in females [6].

Another source of alarm for boys in adolescence may be pubertal gynaecomastia, which is the physiologic enlargement of the glandular breast tissue that occurs in between 4 and 69% of boys [8]. In most boys, the pubertal gynaecomastia regresses substantially or resolves after 1 year. Pathologic gynaecomastia is rare in adolescents, but can occur secondary to certain drugs and tumours that alter the balance of androgens and oestrogens. Overweight teenage boys may have the appearance of breasts due to fatty infiltration of the breast, also known as pseudo-gynaecomastia. When palpated, pseudo-gynaecomastia feels like the adjacent adipose tissue in the anterior axillary fold. Pseudo-gynaecomastia regresses with weight loss [9].

## Trends in pubertal timing
Studies have revealed a worldwide trend towards earlier puberty onset in girls. According to a meta-analysis, the age at thelarche has decreased by about 3 months per decade from 1977 to 2013 [10]. The median age of menarche has also decreased globally [11–13].

Pubertal onset is also trending earlier in boys. In a study conducted in the United States, the mean age for entering puberty was 6 months to 2 years earlier than in past studies. Although there is no clear answer as to why puberty is starting earlier, researchers cite faster gains in weight, changes in nutritional intake, and the presence of endocrine-disrupting chemicals in our food and environment [14–16].

## Sexual and gender development

Sexual and gender development begin early in childhood. Children learn to classify their own and others' sex and develop an understanding of the various aspects of gender [17]. Discussion of sexual and gender development can be multi-faceted, and thus, a set of shared definitions can be useful. According to the World Health Organization:

- Sex refers to the various biological and physiological characteristics of females, males, and intersex people, such as chromosomes, hormones, and reproductive organs [18].
- Gender refers to the characteristics of men and women that are socially constructed, including norms, behaviours, and roles associated with each, as well as the relationship between the genders [18].
- Gender identity refers to a person's deeply felt and individual experience of gender, which may or may not be the same as the person's assigned biological sex at birth [18].
- Sexual orientation refers to the emotional, romantic, or sexual attraction a person feels for another [19].

## Gender dysphoria

Most children identify with the gender that is congruent to the sex assigned at birth and show behaviours that are typical for that gender. However, some children may experience an incongruence between their gender identity and sex assigned at birth, expressing behaviours and preferences, typical for the gender they were not assigned to at birth, and sometimes strongly disliking their biological sex characteristics [17]. The 5th edition of the *Diagnostic and Statistical Manual (DSM) of Mental Disorders* introduces the terminology "gender dysphoria" (GD) to describe the distress caused by this incongruence [20]. Adolescence is a critical time for identity formation and psychosexual development in young people with gender identity concerns. The outcomes of GD in childhood are typically described using the terms persistence and desistence. For most, whether the GD will persist or desist is determined by aged 10–13 years, but some may need more time [21]. As they consider various options, adolescents experiencing gender dysphoria are at an increased risk of mental health issues, including depression and suicide, violence and abuse, eating disorders (EDs), and substance use. Healthcare providers can help these youth and families successfully navigate gender dysphoria issues, providing psychosocial and behavioural support. When indicated, healthcare providers can help to postpone puberty and provide gender-affirming care [22].

## Cross cultural identity development

In today's globalising world, fewer and fewer truly monocultural communities exist, and the traditional way a community defines itself as "'us' versus 'them'" is breaking down. As a result, adolescents rarely grow up experiencing only one culture. In any given day, they can interact with people from diverse cultures, either first-hand or indirectly through traditional media and social media. While this overall is a positive development, the psychological task of forming a cultural identity has become more complex for many adolescents. However, adolescents are more open to new beliefs and behaviours than adults, putting them at the forefront of globalisation [23].

# HEALTH CHALLENGES IN ADOLESCENCE

## Mental health

Depression, anxiety, and other mental health disorders are among the primary causes of illness and disability in the adolescent population with suicide being the fourth leading cause of death among 15–19-year-olds. According to the WHO, one in seven adolescents experiences a mental health disorders [24]. Research suggests that the normal developmental changes that occur during these critical years, including hormonal changes, changes in sleep patterns, pressure to conform with peers, and the exploration of self-concept contribute to the heightened risk of mental illness. Therefore, it is likely that known risks for mental health disorders in childhood, such as genetic predisposition and family risk factors, interact with normal developmental processes in adolescence, triggering the emergence of mental health disorders [25].

Of these disorders, disruptive behaviour disorders and anxiety disorders are the most common. Disruptive behaviour disorders are attention-deficit hyperactivity disorder (ADHD), conduct disorder, and oppositional defiant disorder, while anxiety disorders include diagnoses of social phobia, separation anxiety, panic attacks, generalised anxiety, and obsessive-compulsive disorder [26]. ADHD, characterised by difficulty paying attention and excessive activity with little regard to consequences, occurs in about 5.5% of 10–19-year-olds. Conduct disorder, which involves symptoms of destructive behaviour, occurs in 6.0% of 10–19-year-olds. ADHD can negatively impact an adolescent's education and function. Conduct disorder in adolescence increases the risk of criminal behaviour in adulthood [24].

Anxiety disorders are the most prevalent in adolescents with about 8.2% of 10–19-year-olds experiencing anxiety [24]. Social anxiety disorder, which is characterised by significant and persistent fear of being embarrassed or scrutinised by others, is the prototypical adolescent disorder with a median onset at ages of 13–14 years [25]. For adolescents, peers are the most important socialising influence on behaviour and values as they begin to become increasingly autonomous from their parents. Hence, peer relationships serve as a bridge as adolescents move away from their family unit and towards independent adult functioning. During this crucial phase of social re-orientation and learning, adolescents naturally develop a heightened sense of self-consciousness. This, in turn, increases adolescents' vulnerability for the emergence of social anxiety [27]. Aside from these two groups of disorders, depression also appears to have a higher incidence during the adolescent period, especially among girls [25].

Of great concern, the prevalence of depression and anxiety symptoms among adolescents have doubled during coronavirus disease 2019 (COVID-19), compared with pre-pandemic estimates [28]. School closures and lockdowns disrupted the normal routines and social networks that adolescents developmentally relied on. Preliminary investigations further reveal an increase in self-harm and suicidal behaviour among adolescents during the pandemic [29]. Therefore, it is imperative that healthcare providers prioritise mental health screening in adolescents, providing treatment, guidance, and referrals to mental health services [28].

## Body image and eating disorders

Eating disorders also commonly emerge during adolescence with peak onset between 15 and 19 years. Adolescent girls account for most ED diagnoses, though increasingly more boys are being diagnosed with ED. Internalised beauty standards portrayed by the media cause adolescents to compare their own bodies with the ideal, triggering body image disturbances when the ideal is not achieved. While girls are under pressure to appear thinner, boys also face pressure to have bigger, more muscular bodies [30]. For adolescent girls, weight gain associated with puberty has been linked to the distorted body image, low-self-esteem, symptoms of depression, and the development of EDs [25].

Eating disorders are characterised by abnormal eating behaviours, ranging from restrictive to binging, an unhealthy pre-occupation with food, and often concerns about body weight and shape. The disorders include anorexia nervosa, binge ED, bulimia nervosa, avoidant/restrictive food intake disorder, and several other subtypes and categories outlined by DSM-V. Anorexia nervosa involves restrictive eating behaviour due to a distorted body image and extreme fear of gaining weight. Binge ED is characterised by recurring episodes of eating a large amount a food in short span of time, associated with a sense of lack of control. Bulimia nervosa is marked by similar binge episodes followed by compensatory behaviours to avoid weight gain, like self-induced vomiting or laxative abuse. EDs are associated with significant morbidity and premature mortality, often due to medical complications or suicide [31].

Despite the high prevalence of EDs among adolescents and significant associated medical complications, EDs are still underdiagnosed. An ED should be suspected in an individual of any weight with significant weight loss, growth stunting, pubertal delay, restrictive or binging eating behaviours, recurrent vomiting, excessive exercise, frequent laxative use, or body image concerns. Younger patients are more likely to present with failure to gain expected weight or achieve expected height as opposed to weight loss. Boys and adolescents who are overweight are at risk for delayed diagnosis. Thus, healthcare providers need to be more attentive when dealing with these populations [32]. Though not extensively studied in the adolescent population, screening tools like the ED screen for primary care (EDS-PC) or the SCOFF questionnaire can be used by providers to screen for EDs in adolescents (**Boxes 1.1 and 1.2**) [33].

## Social media use

Social media has become an integral part of adolescents' lives. A cross-national study found that one in three adolescents reported online contact with others via social media almost all the time throughout the day [35,36]. Social media could be viewed as a double-edge sword.

---

**Box 1.1. Eating disorder screen for primary care (EDS-PC) [34]**

- Are you satisfied with your eating patterns?
- Do you ever eat in secret?
- Does your weight affect the way you feel about yourself?
- Have any members of your family suffered with an eating disorder?
- Do you currently suffer with, or have you ever suffered in the past with an eating disorder?

**Box 1.2. SCOFF questionnaire [34]**

- Do you make yourself Sick because you feel uncomfortably full?
- Do you worry you have lost Control over how much you eat?
- Have you recently lost more than One stone (14 lb or 7.7 kg) in a 3-month period?
- Do you believe yourself to be Fat when others say you are thin?
- Would you say that Food dominates your life?

**Box 1.3. Social media screening questions [38]**

All paediatric patients >11 years should be asked the following:

1. Which social media sites and/or apps do you regularly use?
2. How long do you spend on social media sites and/or applications in a typical day?
   - *Concerning response:* >120 min/day
   - *Practical tip:* most smartphones track the total time spent in each application. Ask the patient if they would be willing to follow these instructions to get a more accurate response
   - *iOS instructions:* Settings → Battery → Clock icon → scroll down to "Battery Usage". May also download the applications listed below from the App Store
   - *Android instructions:* will need to download an application that tracks usage. Free options in the Google Play Store include Qualitytime, Break Free, and Checky
3. Do you think you use social media too much?
   - *If yes, ask if they have tried any strategies to remedy it*
4. Does viewing social media increase or decrease your self-confidence?
5. Have you personally experienced cyberbullying, sexting, or an online user asking to have sexual relations with you?
   - *Depending on the patient, the clinician may need to describe what these are*

On one hand, social media allows people to express their opinions and receive social support. However, research also shows a link between social media use and psychological distress in adolescents [37]. Thus, healthcare providers should screen for social media use, just like they would screen for other potentially problematic health behaviours. The American Academy of Paediatrics has suggested potential screening questions, which will allow providers to identify at-risk adolescents and create an opportunity for patient education (**Box 1.3**) [38].

## Substance use

As a result of the imbalance between the socio-emotional system and a cognitive-control system in the adolescent brain, risky behaviours such as smoking, drinking, and illicit drug use often begin in adolescence. Tobacco smoking is the world's leading cause of preventable death and most adult smokers began smoking in adolescence. Globally, roughly 1 in every 10 girls aged 13–15 years and 1 in every 5 boys aged 13–15 years use tobacco, although there are areas where the prevalence is higher [39]. Alcohol drinking among adolescents is another major concern given that it can impair decision-making and increase risky behaviour, leading to injury, violence, and death. Worldwide, more than a quarter of adolescents aged 15–19 years drink alcohol, amounting to 155 million adolescents [40]. Moreover, compared to adults, adolescents are more likely engage in "binge drinking," and consume higher quantities of alcohol per occasion [41]. Magnetic resonance imaging (MRI) studies reveal that alcohol drinking and particularly binge drinking significantly alter the structure of the developing brain, possibly contributing to long-term deficits in learning, memory, and executive function [42,43]. Adolescents using cannabis and other illicit drugs also have been found to develop neurocognitive deficits, leading to behavioural, emotional, and academic problems [40].

Hence, early detection and developmentally sensitive interventions are imperative in addressing substance-associated problems in adolescents. Brief screening tools, such as the Screening to Brief Intervention (S2BI) or the Brief Screener for Tobacco, Alcohol, and Other Drugs (BSTAD), can be used to identify substance use in adolescents. These initial screeners can then be followed up with assessments, like the CRAFFT tool (https://crafft.org), which can further evaluate the level of substance use and severity of functional impairment [44]. After screening, providers can provide brief intervention in the form of motivational interviewing and then refer patients to specialist services and treatment. In motivational interviewing, providers seek to explore the adolescent's motivations for engaging in substance use and intervene accordingly, balancing the adolescent's need for autonomy with reinforcement of healthy behaviours. Research suggests that motivational interviewing is highly efficacious in improving substance use outcomes in adolescents [45].

## Sexual health

While initiation of sexual activity varies widely worldwide, in most regions, adolescents are reaching puberty earlier and often engaging in sexual activity at a younger age. Due to adolescents' propensity for risky behaviours, they are more likely to engage in sexual activity without adequate knowledge and skills regarding safe sex. Moreover, adolescent girls are at a higher risk of sexual coercion, exploitation, and violence, and thus, are more likely to suffer consequences like unintended pregnancy, unsafe abortions, and sexually transmitted infections (STI) [46]. Every year, about 21 million girls aged 15–19 years become pregnant. Pregnancy during adolescence is linked to a higher risk of eclampsia and systemic infections. Babies born to adolescent mothers are more likely to be preterm and have low-birth-weight [47]. Early motherhood also disrupts educational attainment and economic potential. Since there is a significant unmet need for modern contraception among adolescent girls worldwide, there is a high burden of unwanted pregnancies. Consequently, 4.5 million adolescents undergo an abortion every year and 40% of them are performed in unsafe conditions, leading to significant morbidity and mortality [46]. Globally, adolescents have the highest incidence of STIs [48]. Prompt STI treatment is essential because they can facilitate HIV transmission and impact fertility. However, most adolescents do not have access to affordable STI/HIV services [46]. While the incidence of HIV infections has decreased in adolescents, they still account for about 10% of new adult HIV infections, with three-quarters amongst adolescent girls [40].

# THE SSHADESS SCREENING: A STRENGTH-BASED PSYCHOSOCIAL ASSESSMENT

As outlined throughout this chapter, adolescents face unique developmental and health challenges. To identify and address these challenges in our adolescent patients before crises occur, a thorough psychosocial interview should be done by healthcare providers. The SSHADESS (strengths, school, home, activities, drugs, emotions/eating, sexuality, and safety) screening provides a standardised, a strength-based approach to conducting the adolescent psychosocial interview. Building on strengths is the single most important thing you can do to support adolescents through their challenges and prevent them from engaging in high-risk behaviours.

*SSHADESS* represents the following:

- *S* is for *strengths* or positive attributes. Asking adolescents what they perceive as their best abilities is a fascinating way to start a discussion and can be very revealing.
- *S* is for *school or work*. Ask the adolescent about what they enjoy doing in school (or work) and if they are having any specific difficulties. Find out what their future dreams are and ask them to identify who in their life can help them achieve that dream.
- *H* is for *home life*. Where and who does the adolescent live with? Do they feel safe at home?
- *A* is for *activities*. Ask what connects the adolescent to their peers and community, including community service and extracurricular activities. Find out about their sleep, screen time, and social media use.
- *D* is for *diet, drugs, and alcohol use*, plus body image. Ask them about whether they have peers who smoke cigarettes or drink alcohol. Then ask if they have every tried to smoke cigarettes or drink alcohol.
- *E* is for *emotions* (including depression and suicidal thoughts). It is critical to ask adolescents about their mood and whether they have ever self-harmed or felt as if life is not worth living. Please be aware that simply asking the question does not increase a teen's chance of self-injury, but it may be instrumental in identifying a need and providing support.
- *S and S* stand for *sexual health and safety*. Ask who they are attracted to, what their gender identity may be, and how safe they feel in their relationships and community [49].

## CONCLUSION

Adolescence, a critically important and exciting phase of human development, can present unique challenges. A good understanding of these and a systematic but individualised approach is vital in influencing long-term improvements in health outcomes.

## REFERENCES

1. Bitsko R, Claussen A, Lichstein J, Black L. Mental Health Surveillance Among Children – United States, 2013–2019. MMWR Suppl 2022; 71:1–42.
2. Diekema DS. Adolescent brain development and medical decision-making. Pediatrics 2020; 146:S18–S24.
3. Wood CL, Lane LC, Cheetham T. Puberty: Normal physiology (brief overview). Best Pract Res Clin Endocrinol Metab 2019; 33:101265.

4.  Susman E, Houts RM, Steinberg L, et al. Longitudinal Development of Secondary Sexual Characteristics in Girls and Boys Between Ages 9½ and 15½ Years. Arch Pediatr Adolesc Med 2010; 164:166–173.
5.  Muir A. Precocious puberty. Pediatr Rev 2006; 27:373–381.
6.  Biro FM, Chan Y-M. Normal Puberty. In: Duryea TK, Snyder PJ, Geffner ME, Blake D, Hoppin AG (eds). UptoDate. Netherlands: Wolters Kluwer, 2022.
7.  Biro FM, Greenspan LC, Galvez MP, et al. Onset of breast development in a longitudinal cohort. Pediatrics 2013; 132:1019–1027.
8.  Lemaine V, Cayci C, Simmons P, Petty P. Gynecomastia in adolescent males. Semin Plast Surg 2013; 27:56–61.
9.  Taylor SA. Gynecomastia in children and adolescents. In: Blake D, Geffner ME, Torchia MM (eds), UptoDate. Netherlands: Wolters Kluwer, 2022.
10. Eckert-Lind C, Busch AS, Petersen JH, et al. Worldwide Secular Trends in Age at Pubertal Onset Assessed by Breast Development among Girls: A Systematic Review and Meta-analysis. JAMA Pediatr 2020; 174:1–11.
11. Martinez GM. Trends and patterns in menarche in the United States: 1995 through 2013–2017. Natl Health Stat Report 2020; 1–12.
12. Lee MH, Kim SH, Oh M, Lee KW, Park MJ. Age at menarche in Korean adolescents: Trends and influencing factors. Reprod Health 2016; 13:1–7.
13. Garenne M. Trends in age at menarche and adult height in selected African countries (1950–1980). Ann Hum Biol 2020; 47:25–31.
14. Aris IM, Perng W, Dabelea D, et al. Analysis of Early-Life Growth and Age at Pubertal Onset in US Children. JAMA Netw Open 2022; 5:1–14.
15. Nguyen NTK, Fan HY, Tsai MC, et al. Nutrient intake through childhood and early menarche onset in girls: Systematic review and meta-analysis. Nutrients 2020; 12:1–19.
16. Lee JE, Jung HW, Lee YJ, Lee YA. Current evidence for the roles of early-life endocrine disruptors on pubertal timing in girls. Ann Pediatr Endocrinol Metab 2019; 24:78–91.
17. Cohen-Kettenis PT, Klink D. Adolescents with gender dysphoria. Best Pract Res Clin Endocrinol Metab 2015; 29:485–495.
18. World Health Organization. Gender and Health. 2022. https://www.who.int/health-topics/gender#tab=tab_1 (Last accessed 17th January 2023).
19. Campaign HR. Sexual Orientation and Gender Identity Definitions. Published 2022. https://www.hrc.org/resources/sexual-orientation-and-gender-identity-terminology-and-definitions (Last accessed 17th January 2023).
20. Wagner S, Panagiotakopoulos L, Nash R, et al. Progression of gender dysphoria in children and adolescents: A longitudinal study. Pediatrics 2021; 148:1–11.
21. Kaltiala-Heino R, Bergman H, Työläjärvi M, Frisén L. Gender dysphoria in adolescence: current perspectives. Adolesc Health Med Ther 2018; 31–41.
22. Alderman EM, Breuner CC. Unique needs of the adolescent. Pediatrics 2019; 144:e20193150.
23. Jensen LA, Arnett JJ. Going Global: New Pathways for Adolescents and Emerging Adults in a Changing World. J Soc Issues 2012; 68:473–492.
24. World Health Organization. Adolescent Mental Health. Published 2022. https://www.who.int/news-room/fact-sheets/detail/adolescent-mental-health (Last accessed 17th January 2023).
25. Rapee RM, Oar EL, Johnco CJ, et al. Adolescent development and risk for the onset of social-emotional disorders: A review and conceptual model. Behav Res Ther 2019; 123:103501.
26. Long E, Gardani M, McCann M, et al. Mental health disorders and adolescent peer relationships. Soc Sci Med 2020; 253:112973.
27. Leigh E, Clark DM. Understanding Social Anxiety Disorder in Adolescents and Improving Treatment Outcomes: Applying the Cognitive Model of Clark and Wells (1995). Clin Child Fam Psychol Rev 2018; 21:388–414.
28. Racine N, McArthur BA, Cooke JE, et al. Global Prevalence of Depressive and Anxiety Symptoms in Children and Adolescents during COVID-19: A Meta-analysis. JAMA Pediatr 2021; 175:1142–1150.

29. Michaud PA, Michaud L, Mazur A, et al. The Impact of COVID on Adolescent Mental Health, Self-Harm and Suicide: How Can Primary Care Provider Respond? A Position Paper of the European Academy of Pediatrics. Front Pediatr 2022; 10:1–7.

30. Uchôa F, Uchôa N, Daniele T, et al. Influence of the Mass Media and Body Dissatisfaction on the Risk in Adolescents of Developing Eating Disorders. Int J Environ Res Public Heal Artic 2019; 16:1508.

31. Yager J. Eating disorders: Overview of epidemiology, clinical features, and diagnosis. In: Roy-Byrne PP, Solomon D (eds), UptoDate. Netherlands: Wolters Kluwer, 2022.

32. Campbell K, Peebles R. Eating Disorders in Children and Adolescents: State of the Art Review. Pediatrics 2014; 134:582–592.

33. Davidson KW, Barry MJ, Mangione CM, et al. Screening for Eating Disorders in Adolescents and Adults: US Preventive Services Task Force Recommendation Statement. J Am Med Assoc 2022; 327:1061–1067.

34. Kagan S, Melrose C. The SCOFF questionnaire was less sensitive but more specific than the ESP for detecting eating disorders. Evid Based Nurs 2003; 6:118.

35. Boer M, van den Eijnden RJJM, Boniel-Nissim M, et al. Adolescents' Intense and Problematic Social Media Use and Their Well-Being in 29 Countries. J Adolesc Heal 2020; 66:S89–S99.

36. Boniel-Nissim M, van den Eijnden RJJM, Furstova J, et al. International perspectives on social media use among adolescents: Implications for mental and social well-being and substance use. Comput Human Behav 2022; 129.

37. Keles B, McCrae N, Grealish A. A systematic review: the influence of social media on depression, anxiety and psychological distress in adolescents. Int J Adolesc Youth 2020; 25:79–93.

38. Clark DL, Raphael JL, McGuire AL. HEADS[4]: Social media screening in adolescent primary care. Pediatrics 2018; 141:e20173655.

39. Das JK, Salam RA, Arshad A, Finkelstein Y, Bhutta ZA. Interventions for Adolescent Substance Abuse: An Overview of Systematic Reviews. J Adolesc Heal 2016; 59:S61–S75.

40. World Health Organization. Adolescent and young adult health. 2022. https://www.who.int/teams/maternal-newborn-child-adolescent-health-and-ageing/adolescent-and-young-adult-health/resource-bank-for-adolescent-health/who-guidelines. (Last accessed 17th January 2023).

41. Chung T, Creswell KG, Bachrach R, Clark DB, Martin CS. Adolescent Binge Drinking. Alcohol Res 2018; 39:5–15.

42. Cservenka A, Brumback T. The burden of binge and heavy drinking on the brain: Effects on adolescent and young adult neural structure and function. Front Psychol 2017; 8:1111.

43. Feldstein Ewing SW, Sakhardande A, Blakemore SJ. The effect of alcohol consumption on the adolescent brain: A systematic review of MRI and fMRI studies of alcohol-using youth. NeuroImage Clin 2014; 5:420–437.

44. Gray KM, Squeglia LM. Research Review: What have we learned about adolescent substance use? J Child Psychol Psychiatry Allied Discip 2018; 59:618–627.

45. Barnett E, Sussman S, Smith C, Rohrbach LA, Spruijt-Metz D. Motivational Interviewing for Adolescent Substance Use: A Review of the Literature. Addict Behav 2012; 37s:1325–1334.

46. Morris JL, Rushwan H. Adolescent sexual and reproductive health: The global challenges. Int J Gynecol Obstet 2015; 131:S40–S42.

47. World Health Organization. Adolescent Pregnancy. 2022. https://www.who.int/news-room/fact-sheets/detail/adolescent-pregnancy. (Last accessed 17th January 2023).

48. Zheng Y, Yu Q, Lin Y, et al. Global burden and trends of sexually transmitted infections from 1990 to 2019: an observational trend study. Lancet Infect Dis 2022; 22:541–551.

49. Ginsburg KR. The SSHADESS Screen: A Strength-Based Psychosocial Assessment. Reach Teens 2021:139–143.

# Chapter 2

# Technology for adolescent mental health

## Scaling up delivery of evidence-based psychological interventions

*Terry (Theresa) Fleming, Karolina Stasiak, Sally Merry,*
*Mathijs Lucassen, Russell Pine, Liesje Donkin*

## INTRODUCTION

Mental health difficulties are among the most common causes of morbidity and mortality among adolescents, as outlined in Chapter 1 'Adolescent Health'. Mental distress and disorders impact upon day-to-day functioning, including school attainment, peer and family relationships, quality of life, risk-taking and management of other health concerns. Longer-term, adolescent mental health problems predict increased risk of mental and physical health problems and negative outcomes in adulthood.

Paediatricians often have ongoing relationships with young people and their families. They can be the trusted face of medicine and observe changes in functioning and behaviour. Further, adolescent healthcare includes routine screening for common mental health issues (see Chapter 1). On both counts, paediatricians are uniquely placed to detect mental health difficulties and to provide credible advice. However, this begs the question about how and where to access interventions. In many countries, mental health demands outstrip the supply of mental health services and as a result, young people and their families can be left with frustration about a lack of services or can experience dangerous delays.

**Terry (Theresa) Fleming** PhD, Te Herenga Waka, Victoria University of Wellington, New Zealand
Email: terry.fleming@vuw.ac.nz

**Karolina Stasiak** PhD, The University of Auckland, Auckland, New Zealand
Email: k.stasiak@auckland.ac.nz

**Sally Merry** MBChB MD FRANZCP CCAP, The University of Auckland, Auckland, New Zealand
Email: s.merry@auckland.ac.nz

**Mathijs Lucassen** PhD, The Open University, Milton Keynes, UK
Email: mathijs.lucassen@open.ac.uk

**Russell Pine** PhD, Victoria University of Wellington, Wellington, New Zealand
Email: russell.pine@vuw.ac.nz

**Liesje Donkin** PhD PGDipClinPsych, Auckland University of Technology, Auckland, New Zealand
Email: liesje.donkin@aut.ac.nz

Digital innovations offer a promising way forward. Over recent decades, psychological therapies have been translated into computerised or online formats. There is a strong evidence-base for many of these, for example, multiple computerised cognitive behavioural therapy (cCBT) programmes have been shown to have equivalent effects to evidence-based face-to-face therapies [1–3]. However, there are also a plethora of untested apps and programmes [4], and important challenges or questions remain. In this chapter, we outline the opportunities afforded by technology, including current evidence, critical questions, and promising directions.

## BACKGROUND

Estimates prior to the coronavirus disease 2019 (COVID-19) pandemic indicated that one in seven adolescents experienced mental health difficulties [5,6] and these rates appear to be increasing [7] in part exacerbated by the pandemic [8]. Rates of mental health difficulties are higher among adolescents who experience financial hardship [9], are sexual or gender minority [10,11], are indigenous [12,13], and those with chronic or complex medical conditions [14,15]. Talking therapies such as cognitive behavioural therapy (CBT) and acceptance and commitment therapy (ACT) have been shown to be effective for treating mood disorders and anxiety disorders [16–19] including among adolescents with long-term physical conditions [20]. There is some indication that brief interventions may be as effective as more comprehensive programmes [21]. While medications can be effective, generally psychological therapies are the first line of treatment and many guidelines recommend that if medication is used, it is in conjunction with talking therapies [22]. Despite these options, less than one-third of adolescents with diagnosable mental health conditions access treatment [23]. Reasons include a lack of appropriate, convenient or affordable services [24] and social and psychological barriers such as stigma [23,24], limited health literacy [23] and 'help-negating' features of the disorders themselves such as feelings of hopelessness and helplessness [25].

## TECHNOLOGY FOR ADOLESCENT MENTAL HEALTH

### Opportunities afforded by technology

In the face of these challenges, technologies offer important opportunities. Health information, options for help, strategies for dealing with problems and even evidence-based therapies can all be delivered digitally, 24/7, often with low cost for scaling up to large numbers of users. This is potentially transformative, reaching those who would otherwise have limited access to specialist support. Digital interventions can be designed to ensure programme fidelity and provide links to clinical services. They can allow ready translation across languages and adjustments for different settings.

There are four key areas in which digital tools offer promise in adolescent mental health:

1. *Reach:* Digital tools can reach large numbers of people, including those in remote areas, those with limited access to appropriate providers, and those who prefer not to use other options. Although there are 'digital divides' or disparities in access to devices, the internet and relevant programmes, in many cases these are less than divides in access to face-to-face mental health services. In particular, patients from minority identity groups may find it easier to access digital tools tailored for them than to find tailored clinical services in their geographical locality [4,25].

2. *Engagement:* Digital tools offer an 'engagement' potential. While some patients will prefer more traditional face-to-face services, many young people are uncertain or reluctant to engage with mental health professionals and may be more likely to engage with digital options [25,26].

3. *Mechanisms of change*: While many digital tools utilise therapeutic techniques that are established in face-to-face therapies, they can utilise new mechanisms of change, for example, making use of visual imagery and game mechanics to support experiential learning and behaviour change [27,28].

4. *Support existing practice:* Digital tools can also supplement existing practice, for example, gamifying the teaching of social skills, automating routine assessments, or being used alongside face-to-face therapies, for example, to teach core CBT skills and allowing a clinician to focus on individual contexts and personal needs [4].

## Varied technologies and integration with services

The use of technologies for mental health is a diverse and rapidly growing field. The technologies themselves vary widely. They include simple low-cost websites or text messaging interventions which can facilitate help seeking, offer opportunities to communicate with peers or professionals or provide psychoeducation and strategies. They include structured online psychotherapeutic treatments, often offered in a series of modules using video, audio and/or text material and sometimes using game-based or alternative formats. They include apps which may offer specific tools such as a mood diary or a mindfulness intervention, or a full stand-alone treatment [4,25,29]. Other formats include automated chatbots, live interaction functions as well as virtual reality (VR) and augment reality (AR). For example, VR or simulations have been used to address phobias [30] and body dysmorphia [31].

The extent to which technologies are integrated with human support and services also vary. Digital tools can be fully automated self-help interventions, which users can access without referral or the support of a therapist. There are multiple evidence-based self-help tools offering therapeutic components or full evidence-based therapies [32–34]. Fully self-help tools can reach large numbers of people at low cost per user and offer anonymous support. However, these typically have lower completion rates than guided interventions where the user works through a digital programme with a clinician or assistant providing telephone calls, emails or in-person reminders or support [35]. Even brief messages may offer a sense of accountability or support motivation to complete online programmes [35]. Digital tools can also be offered in a blended approach [4], where they are integrated into the primary non-digital therapy process, utilising digital tools for assessments, or to augment the therapeutic process, for example, having a patient completing an online module as homework [36]. Finally, digital tools can be fully integrated within clinical services, such as when video-conferencing is used to enable remote delivery of services [4].

## Use in practice

Hospitals and medical facilities worldwide including Johns Hopkins Medicine and King's College Hospital are using technology-based interventions to support clinical practice, enhance patient communication and information sharing, and provide brief interventions to their patients. Starship, a major children's hospital in New Zealand, is using VR to allow young patient to virtually leave the hospital, connect with the world and alleviate boredom or pain.

Public health and other service providers also support access to digital tools such websites, apps, or e-therapies. Examples include SPARX (Smart, Positive, Active, Realistic, X-factor thoughts) for adolescent depression [27,37] and BRAVE-ONLINE for child and adolescent anxiety [38]. These have been rolled out with government funding in New Zealand and Australia respectively, following robust evaluations [27,38]. Several evidence-based apps to support adolescent mental health are also available such as Sleep Ninja [39]. Other innovative use of gaming technology includes AKL-T01, a game designed for children with ADHD to improve their attentional functioning [40].

## Case study

SPARX (https://www.sparx.org.nz/home) is a seven module cCBT programme delivered in gamified format [27,37]. It was co-developed by researchers and clinicians (authors of this chapter TF, KS, SM and ML together with Dr Mathew Shepherd), young people, cultural advisors and a game development company, Metia Interactive. SPARX uses a 'bicentric frame of reference' where a guide (virtual therapist) introduces the game and each module [27]. After 'speaking' to the guide, users enter a fantasy world where they complete quests and solve puzzles which provide non-threatening and autonomy-enhancing ways to discover insights and rehearse skills. For example:

- Practicing making decisions, testing them out and trying again if they do not work.
- Finding and releasing a 'bird of hope' who usually, but does not always, accompany the user thereafter; and,
- 'Shooting' and categorising 'gloomy negative automatic thoughts'.

At the end of game-play users return to the guide to consolidate their learning, e.g. via the use of playful quizzes and to reflect on what they will try in real life.

SPARX was not inferior to treatment as usual in a large randomised controlled trial (RCT) [27], and indigenous Māori young people found it to be a useful intervention [41]. It has been adapted for sexual minority youth and other under-served populations [42–44], although versions have been unappealing with young people in a youth justice and some alternative education settings [37,44]. At the time of writing SPARX is freely available to those with a New Zealand IP address and it can be purchased in Japan. There are various trials of SPARX and developments from it, including a prevention focussed version [44–46] and a refined version for indigenous Nunavut young people in Canada [47].

---

**CASE EXAMPLE**

### Introducing computerised therapy in clinical practice

- Lachlan, a 13-year-old cystic fibrosis (CF) patient, is reviewed regularly in a paediatric respiratory clinic. Although Lachlan and his family had previously managed Lachlan's CF well, his general adherence to treatment had started to deteriorate. During an appointment, it was apparent that Lachlan had been struggling with feeling different from his peers, with concerns about how his body looked and missing out on some peer activities. He was frustrated with his parents' 'hovering' over him and his lack of independence. His mother had noticed that he seemed more withdrawn and had been trying to get him 'out of the house more'. Despite Lachlan having negative thoughts, he did not meet the criteria for an assessment at his local mental health service and he did not want to talk to a therapist

*Continues opposite*

- His paediatrician, recognising that it was important to address these negative beliefs, began to explore alternative treatment options. She discovered an online evidence-based self-help therapy. At a follow-up appointment, she showed Lachlan the programme, and they started the first module together during the appointment. Lachlan agreed to complete the rest of the programme before their next appointment a month later. Together, Lachlan and his paediatrician spoke to Lachlan's mother and Lachlan smugly told his mother that his treatment plan was to play an online game
- At their next appointment, Lachlan reported that despite his doubts, the programme had helped. Specifically, he found that recognising certain negative thoughts as 'things to beat' rather than absolute truths about himself was helpful. He also reported that he had been able to talk to his mother and friends about his difficulties through demonstrating the programme to them (which he found easier than talking about what was going on directly)

## Evidence base

Evidence for technology-based interventions is growing rapidly. A 2021 review, for example, identified 246 systematic reviews of digital interventions related to mental health and wellbeing [29]. Diverse therapeutic approaches, differing technologies and varied levels of clinical integration mean that it is of limited value to endeavour to attempt to synthesise the effectiveness of all digital technologies for mental health in single combined analyses, however, there are robust randomised controlled trials of specific digital programmes, and multiple systematic reviews and meta-analyses identifying that self-help and guided cCBT programmes are effective for mental health problems including depression [e.g. 1,3] anxiety [e.g. 2,3] and somatic disorders [e.g. 48].

At the same time, many commercially available apps, websites and digital therapies are developed with no clinical guidance or evidence base. For example, in a recent review, only 3.4% of apps available on common platforms provided evidence of effectiveness [4].

In the face of this rapidly changing environment, recommendations or endorsement by reputable groups is valuable. Some professional and academic groups offer reviews of the evidence or endorsements for specific tools. For example, see National Health Service wellbeing app guidance, One Mind Psyberguide or the National Registry of Evidence-based Programs and Practices (NREPP) in the United States of America. Several guidelines have been developed to support the adoption of technology into clinical practice, including The National Institute for Health and Care Excellence (NICE) Evidence Standards Framework (ESF) for Digital Health Technologies [49], and the World Health Organization's Recommendations on Digital Interventions for Health System Strengthening [50].

## Challenges

Aside from the plethora of rapidly changing options and evidence, challenges in the use of technology-based interventions include high attrition or drop-out rates in many digital tools [51] and uncertainty from both patients and providers.

Patients may expect face-to-face support and require assurance that digital tools are effective. For some groups, access to devices, perceived relevance of digital tools or knowing which tools to trust are problematic. Likewise, clinicians may be unsure about the effectiveness of digital tools, or have concerns about suitability or safety [52]. There is often the assumption that patients would not want to use technology-based interventions [52] despite evidence that many patients consider technology-based interventions to be acceptable or even, for some, preferable [e.g. 37,53,54]. Clinician attitudes are important: recommendations or 'prescribing' by clinicians has been shown to influence behaviour. However, this approach is likely to require access to up-to-date resources and training.

# CONCLUSION

Technology-based interventions are a rapidly growing and evolving area driven by demand, pressure on health systems and by opportunities afforded via technology. Technology-based interventions can be used to extend the reach of evidence-based interventions and to offer choice and flexibility to users. Tools have been developed for diverse populations and for varied physical and mental health conditions, and more can be expected each year. The growing body of data supporting the evidence and acceptability of technology-based interventions provides assurance that these tools can be adopted into practice, improving opportunities to address important health needs at scale.

# REFERENCES

1.  Luo C, Sanger N, Singhal N, et al. A comparison of electronically-delivered and face to face cognitive behavioural therapies in depressive disorders: A systematic review and meta-analysis. EClinicalMedicine 2020; 24:100442.
2.  Podina IR, Mogoase C, David D, Szentagotai A, Dobrean A. A meta-analysis on the efficacy of technology mediated CBT for anxious children and adolescents. J Rational-Emotive Cogn Behav Ther 2016; 34:31–50.
3.  Wickersham A, Barack T, Cross L, Downs J. Computerized cognitive behavioral therapy for treatment of depression and anxiety in adolescents: Systematic review and meta-analysis. J Med Internet Res 2022; 24:e29842.
4.  Marshall JM, Dunstan DA, Bartik W. The digital psychiatrist: In search of evidence-based apps for anxiety and depression. Front Psychiatry 2019; 10:e831.
5.  Institute of Health Metrics and Evaluation. Global Health Data Exchange (GHDx). 2023; Available from http://ghdx.healthdata.org/gbd-results-tool?params=gbd-api-2019-permalink/380dfa3f2663 9cb711d908d9a119ded2 [Last accessed 19th January 2023].
6.  Polanczyk GV, Salum GA, Sugaya LS, Caye A, Rohde LA. Annual research review: A meta-analysis of the worldwide prevalence of mental disorders in children and adolescents. J Child Psychol Psychiatry 2015; 56:345–365.
7.  World Health Organization. World mental health report: Transforming mental health for all. Geneva: WHO, 2022.
8.  Ma L, Mazidi M, Li K, et al. Prevalence of mental health problems among children and adolescents during the COVID-19 pandemic: A systematic review and meta-analysis. J Affect Disord 2021; 293:78–89.
9.  Deighton J, Lereya ST, Casey P, et al. Prevalence of mental health problems in schools: poverty and other risk factors among 28 000 adolescents in England. Br J Psychiatry 2019; 215:565–567.
10. Lucassen MF, Stasiak K, Samra R, Frampton CM, Merry SN. Sexual minority youth and depressive symptoms or depressive disorder: A systematic review and meta-analysis of population-based studies. Aust N Z J Psychiatry 2017; 51:774–787.
11. Russell ST, Fish JN. Mental health in lesbian, gay, bisexual, and transgender (LGBT) youth. Annu Rev Clin Psychol 2016; 12:465–487.
12. Azzopardi PS, Sawyer SM, Carlin JB, et al. Health and wellbeing of Indigenous adolescents in Australia: a systematic synthesis of population data. The Lancet 2018; 391:766–782.
13. Harder HG, Rash J, Holyk T, Jovel E, Harder K. Indigenous youth suicide: a systematic review of the literature. Pimatisiwin: J Aborigin Indigen Commun Health 2012; 10:125–142.
14. Pinquart M, Shen Y. Depressive symptoms in children and adolescents with chronic physical illness: An updated meta-analysis. J Pediatr Psychol 2011; 36:375–384.

15. Cobham VE, Hickling A, Kimball H, et al. Systematic review: Anxiety in children and adolescents with chronic medical conditions. J Am Acad Child Adolesc Psychiatry 2020; 59:595–618.
16. Zhou X, Hetrick SE, Cuijpers P, et al. Comparative efficacy and acceptability of psychotherapies for depression in children and adolescents: A systematic review and network meta-analysis. World Psychiatry 2015; 14:207–222.
17. Warwick H, Reardon T, Cooper P, et al. Complete recovery from anxiety disorders following cognitive behavior therapy in children and adolescents: A meta-analysis. Clin Psychol Rev 2017; 52:77–91.
18. Wang Z, Whiteside SPH, Sim L, et al. Comparative effectiveness and safety of cognitive behavioral therapy and pharmacotherapy for childhood anxiety disorders: A systematic review and meta-analysis. JAMA Pediatr 2017; 171:1049–1056.
19. Baker HJ, Lawrence PJ, Karalus J, Creswell C, Waite P. The effectiveness of psychological therapies for anxiety disorders in adolescents: A meta-analysis. Clin Child Fam Psychol Rev 2021; 24:765–782.
20. Thabrew H, Stasiak K, Hetrick SE, et al. Psychological therapies for anxiety and depression in children and adolescents with long-term physical conditions. Cochrane Database Syst Rev 2018; 12:1–164.
21. Öst LG, Ollendick TH. Brief, intensive and concentrated cognitive behavioral treatments for anxiety disorders in children: A systematic review and meta-analysis. Behav Res Ther 2017; 97:134–145.
22. National Institute for Health and Care Excellence, Depression in children and young people: Identification and management NICE guideline [NG134]. London: NICE, 2019.
23. Radez J, Reardon T, Creswell C, et al. Why do children and adolescents (not) seek and access professional help for their mental health problems? A systematic review of quantitative and qualitative studies. Eur Child Adolesc Psychiatry 2021; 30:183–211.
24. Reardon T, Harvey K, Baranowska M, et al. What do parents perceive are the barriers and facilitators to accessing psychological treatment for mental health problems in children and adolescents? A systematic review of qualitative and quantitative studies. Eur Child Adolesc Psychiatry 2017; 26:623–647.
25. Fleming T, Sutcliffe K, Dewhirst M, et al. Digital tools for mental health and wellbeing: Opportunities and impact. Findings from the literature and community research. Wellington: Te Hiringa Hauora Health Promotion Agency, 2021.
26. Fleming T, Sutcliffe K, Lucassen M, Pine R, Donkin L. Serious games and gamification in clinical psychology. In: Asmundson GJG (ed.), Comprehensive Clinical Psychology. Amsterdam: Elsevier, 2022; 77–90.
27. Merry SN, Stasiak K, Shepherd M. The effectiveness of SPARX, a computerised self-help intervention for adolescents seeking help for depression: randomised controlled non-inferiority trial. BMJ 2012; 344:e2598.
28. Pine R, Te Morenga L, Olson M, Fleming T. Development of a casual video game (Match Emoji) with psychological well-being concepts for young adolescents. Digital Health 2021; 7:1–9.
29. De Witte NAJ, Joris S, Van Assche E, Van Daele T. Technological and digital interventions for mental health and wellbeing: An overview of systematic reviews. Front Digital Health 2021; 23:e754337.
30. Botella C, Osma J, Garcia-Palacios A, Quero S, Baños RS. Treatment of flying phobia using virtual reality: Data from a 1-year follow-up using a multiple baseline design. Clin Psychol Psychother 2004; s11:311–323.
31. Gutiérrez-Maldonado J, Ferrer-García M, Dakanalis A, Riva G. Virtual reality: Applications to eating disorders. In: Agras WS, Robinson R (eds), The Oxford Handbook of Eating Disorders. Oxford: Oxford University Press, 2018; 470–491.
32. Bennett SD, Cuijpers P, Ebert DD, et al. Practitioner review: Unguided and guided self-help interventions for common mental health disorders in children and adolescents: a systematic review and meta-analysis. J Child Psychol Psychiatry 2019; 60:828–847.
33. Moshe I, Terhorst Y, Paganini S, et al. Digital interventions for the treatment of depression: A meta-analytic review. Psychol Bulletin 2021; 147:1–38.
34. Lecomte T, Potvin S, Corbière M, et al. Mobile apps for mental health issues: Meta-review of meta-analyses. JMIR MHealth UHealth 2020; 8:e17458.
35. Cuijpers P, Donker T, van Straten A, Li J, Andersson G. Is guided self-help as effective as face-to-face psychotherapy for depression and anxiety disorders? A systematic review and meta-analysis of comparative outcome studies. Psychol Med 2010; 40:1943–1957.

36. Donkin L, Fleming T. Computerized cognitive behavioural therapy and clinical practice. In: Wilson H (ed.), Digital Delivery of Mental Health Therapies. London: Jessica Kingsley, 2022.

37. Fleming T, Lucassen M, Stasiak K, Sutcliffe K, Merry S. Technology Matters: SPARX – computerised cognitive behavioural therapy for adolescent depression in a game format. Child Adolesc Mental Health, 2021; 26:92–94.

38. March S, Spence SH, Donovan CL, Kenardy JA. Large-scale dissemination of internet-based cognitive behavioral therapy for youth anxiety: Feasibility and acceptability study. J Med Internet Res 2018; 20:e9211.

39. Werner-Seidler A, Wong Q, Johnston L, et al. Pilot evaluation of the Sleep Ninja: a smartphone application for adolescent insomnia symptoms. BMJ Open 2019; 9:e026502.

40. Kollins SH, DeLoss DJ, Cañadas E, et al. A novel digital intervention for actively reducing severity of paediatric ADHD (STARS-ADHD): a randomised controlled trial. Lancet Digital Health 2020; 2:e168–e178.

41. Shepherd M, Merry S, Lambie I, Thompson A. Indigenous adolescents' perception of an eMental Health Program (SPARX): exploratory qualitative assessment. JMIR Serious Games 2018; 6:e8752.

42. Lucassen MFG, Merry SN, Hatcher S, Frampton CMA. Rainbow SPARX: A novel approach to addressing depression in sexual minority youth. Cogn Behav Pract 2015; 22:203–216.

43. Lucassen MF, Stasiak K, Fleming T, et al. Computerized cognitive behavioural therapy for gender minority adolescents: Analysis of the real-world implementation of SPARX in New Zealand. Austral N Z J Psychiatry 2021; 55:874–882.

44. Fleming TM, Gillham B, Bavin LM, et al. SPARX-R computerized therapy among adolescents in youth offenders' program: step-wise cohort study. Inter Intervent 2019; 18:e100287.

45. Fleming TM, Stasiak K, Moselen E, et al. Revising computerized therapy for wider appeal among adolescents: Youth perspectives on a revised version of SPARX. Front Psychiatry 2019; 10:e802.

46. Perry Y, Werner-Seidler A, Calear A, et al. Preventing depression in final year secondary students: School-based randomized controlled trial. J Med Inter Res 2017; 19:e8241.

47. Thomas A, Bohr Y, Hankey J, et al. How did Nunavummiut youth cope during the COVID-19 pandemic? A qualitative exploration of the resilience of Inuit youth leaders involved in the I-SPARX project. Int J Circumpolar Health 2022; 81:e2043577.

48. Vigerland S, Lenhard F, Bonnert M, et al. Internet-delivered cognitive behavior therapy for children and adolescents: a systematic review and meta-analysis. Clin Psychol Rev 2016; 50:1–10.

49. National Institute for Health and Care Excellence. Evidence Standards Framework (ESF) for Digital Health Technologies (Corporate document [ECD7]). 2018. Available from https://www.nice.org.uk/corporate/ecd7 (Last accessed 19th January 2023).

50. WHO guideline: recommendations on digital interventions for health system strengthening. Geneva: World Health Organization, 2019. Licence: CC BY-NC-SA 3.0 IGO.

51. Fleming T, Bavin L, Lucassen M, et al. Beyond the trial: systematic review of real-world uptake and engagement with digital self-help interventions for depression, low mood, or anxiety. J Med Internet Res 2018; 20:e9275.

52. Mol M, van Genugten C, Dozeman E, et al. Why uptake of blended internet-based interventions for depression is challenging: A qualitative study on therapists' perspectives. J Clin Med 2019; 9:91.

53. McDermott E, Hughes E, Rawlings V. Queer futures final report: Understanding lesbian, gay, bisexual and trans (LGBT) adolescents' suicide, self-harm and help-seeking behaviour. Lancaster: Lancaster University, 2016.

54. Liverpool S, Mota CP, Sales C et al. Engaging children and young people in digital mental health interventions: Systematic review of modes of delivery, facilitators, and barriers. J Med Internet Res 2020; 22:e16317.

# Chapter 3

# Adolescent gynaecology and breast health – updates from a paediatric perspective

*Heather Brown, Seema Seetharam*

## INTRODUCTION

Adolescent gynaecology consists of patients presenting with adult type symptoms manifesting in children going through an emotionally and physiologically turbulent time. The key focus for any clinician working within this clinical area is to acknowledge the complexities of the patients, to approach the clinical issues holistically and continually endeavour to communicate with the patients on an appropriate level so as to ensure that they stay engaged with their clinician and parents.

## CONSULTATION

Adolescent gynaecology patients are often seen in a children's clinic or hospital setting. While this is usually better than being seen in an adult setting it is not ideal as the toys, children's furniture and decorations may seem incongruous and inappropriate for a consultation related to gynaecological symptoms for a nervous adolescent who is feeling anxious and embarrassed about talking to a clinician about their symptoms. Acknowledging the children's environment and that it is not in keeping with their age can often be helpful.

Parents nearly always accompany their adolescent children, and their support and input are of great value; however, it is important to engage with the girl herself, listen and hear her concerns and her description of how she is experiencing her symptoms and to determine what are her priorities with regard to her symptoms and her preferences in management of her symptoms. At the first consultation it is useful to check with the adolescent regarding their choice of pronouns as this can open up lesbian, gay, bisexual, and transgender, queer and/or questioning individuals (LGBTQ) + discussions and disclosures.

**Heather Brown** MBBCh PhD MRCOG, Consultant Obstetrician and Gynaecologist, Labour Ward Lead, Royal Sussex County Hospital, Honorary Senior Clinical Lecturer, Brighton and Sussex Medical School, Brighton, UK
Email: heather.brown27@nhs.net.

**Seema Seetharam** MBBS MRCS FRCS FEBS Consultant Oncoplastic, Aesthetic and Reconstructive Breast Surgeon, Dartford and Gravesham NHS Trust, Dartford, UK
Email: seemaseetharam@nhs.net

Unlike adult patients attending a gynaecologist appointment, adolescents will not have experienced any form of gynaecological examination and therefore a careful and detailed explanation is the first step. This should include showing the instruments such as speculum, swabs, and where the examination will take place and what clothing they will need to remove, this can be limited to underwear/lower body clothing. Privacy and dignity are always important for gynaecological examinations and particularly for adolescents. Not all symptoms will require an examination and the examination can be scheduled for another day to give the adolescent the opportunity to feel more prepared.

Parents may have different expectations of the outcome of the appointment especially related to treatment. For example, adolescent girls may be keen to have a hormonal treatment for their menstrual symptoms and also for contraceptive needs which they may not have disclosed to their parents. Keeping parents and the adolescent engaged with each other as well as with the consultation and treatment suggestions will improve their satisfaction with the appointment and increase the likelihood of compliance with treatment.

While parents or a family member usually accompany adolescent patients it is important to be clear during introductions regarding whom is present. Children in care may be accompanied by their care worker or foster parent. Consent regarding the accompanying person being present during discussions and examinations should not be assumed and confidentiality needs to be a priority. Chaperones can be used if there is no appropriate person present or the appointment can be rescheduled for a time when an appropriate person can be present. Adolescent patients can sometimes attend alone, in this situation explore whether they understand the topics that will be discussed (e.g. gynaecological symptoms) and give the option to re-schedule the appointment. They may also attend with a friend, also an adolescent which warrants explaining the nature of the topics to be discussed and whether they feel comfortable having their friend present or whether they would like to return with a parent or someone else on another day.

Consent in this age group, if <16 years of age, should be in line with Gillick competency and using the Fraser guidelines for consent to treatment. While Gillick competency was initially described only in relation to contraception in girls under the age of 16 years, its principles can be applicable to other forms of gynaecological care [1].

It is usual for adolescent patients to have researched their symptoms and potential investigations and diagnoses online, including social media, social influencers and it is important to listen to what they have found out thus far; being dismissive of information that they have accessed online or via social media is not helpful and is not in keeping with current methods of learning that adolescents are accessing. Instead suggesting helpful Apps, and other online tools and resources will help to engage the adolescent more fully in their care. For example, most major smartphones have their own free health Apps which include menstrual calendars and gynaecological symptom trackers. The UK-NHS has a confidential resource for health advice for adolescents called #NHS.Go and Brook.org.uk is a UK-based charity for adolescent contraception and sexual health; both are a good online resource.

## HEAVY PERIODS

During adolescence menstrual difficulties are common and have a significant impact on young girls including being a major cause of school absences. Most adolescent gynaecology clinics describe that up to 30% of referrals to the clinic are due to menstrual difficulties [2].

Typically, a girl will experience menarche followed by a few periods which are unproblematic but are then followed by a phase of painful, heavy, long periods which can last for a few years. The heavy periods are often associated with other symptoms of nausea, fainting (usually vasovagal secondary to clots passing through the cervix) and sometimes changes in bowel habits. The physiological background is anovulatory cycles interspersed with ovulatory cycles and appears to be a developmental phase which improves once the cycles all become ovulatory.

Investigations typically include pelvic ultrasound and full blood count and other investigations as guided by the patient history and clinical examination, for example, clotting studies in the presence of other symptoms of bleeding disorder. Investigations including pelvic ultrasound rarely identify any pathology [3] and therefore a pragmatic treatment approach would be to manage the symptoms and only investigate those whose symptoms do not respond to usual treatment. Parents and girls themselves may not be keen to start treatment without a diagnosis or exclusion of pathology with investigations, hence a pelvic ultrasound would be the main investigation.

Treatment starts with mefenamic acid and tranexamic acid and then the combined oral contraceptive (COC), which can be taken continuously until break through bleeding and then re-started 5 days after the onset of the breakthrough bleed. If there are contraindications to the COC, then a progesterone only pill can be effective in causing amenorrhoea. In very young girls, that is under 12 years or within a year of their menarche there is no available evidence and therefore we usually would delay starting the COC in such girls. In this age group, progesterone tablets can be used during the period to reduce the heaviness of the periods without inhibiting ovulation. Current guidance is for the COC to be taken each day for three packets in a row, a 4-day break and then re-start or else continuously until breakthrough bleeding occurs, a 5-day break and then re-start [4].

A family history of similar period problems may be present which is difficult to interpret – is this truly familial or it is attributable to the typical and common heavy periods of adolescence? There may also be overlap with a family history of endometriosis. This is also difficult to interpret as the girl may go onto develop endometriosis in line with her family history, but during adolescence her symptoms may just be related to being an adolescent.

Another cause of heavy menstrual bleeding may be related to pregnancy. The episode of bleeding may prompt the first disclosure by the adolescent of them being sexually active (this can include non-consensual sex) and their fears concerning pregnancy. Early pregnancy units and maternity services will provide management, ideally with specialised teenage pregnancy teams and may include safeguarding and child protection.

Lastly, infections can cause heavy bleeding or irregular bleeding, most of which are sexually transmitted infections and should be managed within young people's sexual health clinics for the appropriate testing and sexual health education.

## Dysmenorrhoea and abdominal pain

Adolescent periods are typically very painful as well as heavy in volume. The pain typically precedes the onset of bleeding, continues during the period and then sometimes stops a day or two after the bleeding has ended. Similar to the heavy menstrual bleeding, this seems to be a developmental stage associated with anovulatory cycles and often improves as the girl gets older. It is also common to get mid-cycle pain, on one side of the lower abdomen which is as a result of ovulation – ovulation pain. Investigations for heavy menstrual bleeding will include identifying and excluding causes of abdominal pain;

there is a very low pick-up rate for pathology in this age group. Management will follow the same approach as for the heavy menstrual bleeding that is mefenamic acid for analgesia and contraceptive methods to reduce the number of periods/intentional amenorrhoea.

## Primary amenorrhoea

Menarche is one component of reaching sexual maturity, the others being thelarche (breast development) and adrenarche (appearance of pubic and axillary hair, body odour and acne). The steps in sexual maturation are described in Tanner stages 1–5 (see **Table 3.1**). A delay in starting their periods is a common cause for concern for adolescent girls and their parents, particularly once all of their peers have started their periods. The traditional definition of primary amenorrhoea is the lack of menses by the age of 16 years. This has been revised and now investigation would be warranted if: there is no menses by the age of 15 years, even with normal growth and the presence of secondary sexual characteristics; no menses within 3 years of thelarche; no menses by the age of 14 years in the absence of a growth spurt and no development of secondary sexual characteristics; no menses by the age of 14 years with signs of hirsutism or a history of an eating disorder or excessive exercise (hypothalamic cause). Investigations would include blood test to look at the levels of follicle-stimulating hormone (FSH), luteinising hormone (LH) and oestradiol, pelvic ultrasound once a clinical examination has been carried out to identify the presence or absence of secondary sexual characteristics and other clinical signs such as acne, hirsutism, height and weight (see **Figure 3.1**). Very often no cause is identified, the girl and her parents can be reassured and menarche starts spontaneously.

True primary amenorrhoea is rare and may be due to a variety of different causes – endocrine, chromosomal, congenital and acquired. The endocrine causes can be divided into those that present with raised serum gonadotropins or those with normal or low gonadotropins (see **Figure 3.1**). Many of these rare causes of primary amenorrhoea (see **Table 3.2**) should be referred to specialist centres for multi-disciplinary care to include medical, surgical, and psychological care.

## Secondary amenorrhoea

Secondary amenorrhoea is a more challenging situation in adolescents than primary amenorrhoea. As the girl has already had a menarche and a number of periods, we can be assured that the anatomical structures involved in menstruation are able to

| Table 3.1  Tanner stages/sexual maturity for girls | | |
|---|---|---|
| Stage | Breast | Pubic hair |
| 1 | Elevation of papilla of breast | No pubic hair |
| 2 | Elevation of the breast and papilla to form breast bud | Sparse, downy or straight hair along labia |
| 3 | Further enlargement of breast and areola | Darker, coarser, curly hair |
| 4 | Secondary mound above level of breast | Adult hair type spreads over the mons pubis |
| 5 | Mature breast and recession of areola to general contour of the breast | Adult-type hair in quality and quantity, spreads to inner surface of thighs |

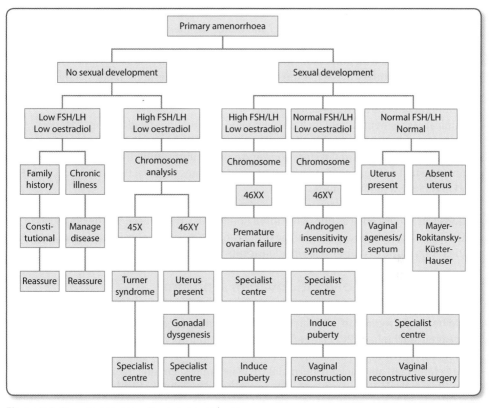

**Figure 3.1** Investigations in primary amenorrhoea.

(FSH, follicle-stimulating hormone; LH, luteinising hormone)

| Table 3.2. Causes of primary amenorrhoea | |
|---|---|
| **Category** | **Diagnosis** |
| Increased serum gonadotropins | • Premature ovarian insufficiency<br>• XX or XY gonadal dysgenesis<br>• Turner's syndrome<br>• Irradiation/cytotoxic therapy<br>• Autoimmune/infectious |
| Normal or low serum gonadotropins | • Constitutional delay<br>• Panhypopituitarism<br>• Isolated gonadotropin deficiency<br>• Kallman's syndrome (with anosmia)<br>• Hypothalamic dysfunction<br>• Chronic illness<br>• Eating disorders/excess exercise/stress<br>• CNS tumours/lesions/malformations<br>• Hypothyroidism<br>• Hyperprolactinaemia, i.e. adenoma, medication<br>• Syndromes with hypo-hypo Prader–Willi, Lawrence–Moon's syndrome, Bardet Bield |
| Other conditions | • Anatomic abnormalities (Müllerian agenesis, cervical agenesis, transverse septum, and imperforate hymen)<br>• Androgen insensitivity syndrome<br>• Noonan's syndrome |

function and hence the cause is to be found within the hypothalamic-pituitary-ovarian axis (HPO axis) which controls ovulation and hence the menstrual cycle. The presence or absence of symptoms can give direction towards a cause, for example, symptoms of hyperandrogenism with polycystic ovarian syndrome (PCOS), headaches and visual field changes with a pituitary mass. It is important to ask direct questions about symptoms of hyperandrogenism as make-up and hair removal techniques may mean that these symptoms are not obvious as clinical signs.

Clinical assessment should include height and weight. Investigations for secondary amenorrhoea should include blood tests to assess the HPO axis – FSH, LH, prolactin, oestradiol, progesterone and testosterone and a pelvic ultrasound. If there are associated symptoms such as headaches, galactorrhoea and changes to visual fields then add an MRI head to exclude a pituitary mass.

Polycystic ovarian syndrome as a cause of secondary amenorrhoea is a more difficult diagnosis in adolescence as one of the three Rotterdam Criteria used for the diagnosis of PCOS [5], polycystic appearances of the ovary can be a normal appearance for adolescent ovaries. This is due to many cycles in adolescents being anovulatory.

## Management of polycystic ovarian syndrome

Girls with PCOS often have a raised BMI which means that the focus of management would be weight reduction, often needing the support of specialist dietary services. As with all age groups who have PCOS, weight reduction is often very challenging and requires support and encouragement from the clinicians. Identifying a realistic weight loss goal is more helpful than aiming for a 'normal BMI' which may seem unachievable to the girl with PCOS. Research shows us that even a 5% reduction in weight can result in the resumption of ovulation and menstrual cycles.

The other component of management of PCOS in girls who are still having periods, but the periods are troublesome, would be the use of a contraceptive pill, combined or progesterone only depending on the girls' weight and any other medical history [6].

Adolescence is a life stage that can contain significant sources of life stress such as school examinations, bullying (including social media bullying), engaging in sports and dance at highly competitive levels all of which can result in amenorrhoea at a hypothalamic level. Concerns about body image are common, prompting over excessive exercise, eating disorders and conversely obesity. Parents and families may be unaware of any problems. Offering to talk to the girl on her own may be helpful as are closed questions: instead of asking 'do you over-exercise?' ask 'how many hours per week do you exercise?'; change 'do you eat healthily?' to 'can you take me through what you would eat in a typical day?' Or 'I would like you to use an App between now and your next appointment to keep a diary of all the food you eat in a week'. Sometimes the questions are effective by raising the possibility of a problem.

If secondary amenorrhoea persists without a clear cause then using a progesterone challenge to generate a period can prompt a return to a normal cycle. A progesterone challenge involves taking oral norethisterone tablets for 19 days, on stopping the progesterone a period will commence. Alternatively, a combined oral contraceptive can be used to provide exogenous oestradiol and to generate regular withdrawal bleeds for 6–12 months.

## Intentional amenorrhoea

Within any adolescent gynaecology service there will be a small cohort of girls who present seeking intentional amenorrhoea. This group includes girls with medical conditions, mental health problems, mood and behavioural issues and girls with special care needs that mean that they are unable to manage their own toilet needs which once they begin to menstruate includes managing the practicalities of their periods.

There are many conditions that that are affected by the hormonal peaks and troughs within the menstrual cycle, the most frequently presenting being epileptic (and non-epileptic) seizures and migraines. In order to flatten the peaks and troughs of hormonal levels in these girls contraceptive medication can be prescribed to inhibit ovulation. Epileptic medication may impact on the contraceptive efficacy of the medication which is important to be aware of in girls who are sexually active. While the contraceptive efficacy is affected the cycle control efficacy seems to be less markedly affected and therefore this may not be a problem in girls who are younger and not sexually active.

Migraine sufferers often experience an exacerbation of symptoms pre-menstrually and also benefit from medication to inhibit ovulation. Migraine, particularly with aura, is a contraindication for the combined contraceptive pills and therefore a progesterone only pill should be used or else a long-acting reversible contraceptive (LARC) such as the implant or an intrauterine system [7].

Parents and carers of girls in care with special needs describe a deterioration in mood and behavioural problems pre-menstrually. Contraceptives can again be used, taking note of other medical conditions but also other specific to that girl's special needs, e.g. whether the girl will tolerate taking tablets daily, tolerate having a patch on their skin or whether they will peel it off, tolerate a sub-dermal implant or whether they would try to self-remove.

Carers and parents of girls with significant medical co-morbidities which mean they are unable to manage their own toilet hygiene and subsequent menstrual hygiene may request methods to ensure amenorrhoea. There may also be concerns around dysmenorrhoea being particularly distressing to girls who are unable to understand the physiological experience of menstruation. The issue of consent needs to be carefully explored as well as physical co-morbidities including immobility which would result in the progesterone preparations being the most appropriate, excluding the depot injections due to their impact on bone density.

Parents of this group of girls experience a sense of grief and loss when their child starts their menarche as it is a physical sign of progression to adulthood that will not be matched with any other steps towards independent living or adulthood.

# TRANSGENDER PATIENTS

During transition and while living as their new gender, transgender males may be referred to achieve amenorrhoea using hormonal contraceptives including LARCs. Other components of transitioning would be provided by referral to a specialist transgender centre, however, there can be long waits to be seen in such services hence an adolescent gynaecology service can provide interim care. Understanding the issues around transitioning and acknowledgement and use of the correct pronouns is of great importance and should be guided by the young persons' choices.

## Vulval appearance

During puberty there are a number of physiological changes which result in dramatic changes in physical appearance as the girl child moves into adolescence and ultimately into adulthood. Most of these changes are anticipated by girls such as breast development and axillary and pubic hair. However, there is less awareness about the changes in the appearance of the vulva and vagina which includes an increase in size of the labia and deposition of subcutaneous fat over the mons pubis. These changes can become a cause for concern and anxiety for girls. Girls of this age are typically shy about their bodies and will avoid being seen naked by their parents, or peers even in sports changing room settings and hence they do not have a reference range of normal vulval appearance. This applies to their mothers or older sisters who equally have little understanding of the wide range of normal vulval appearance and may also apply to primary care practitioners once their opinion is sought. Hence, girls are referred to a specialist service which compounds their concern that the appearance of their vulva is abnormal. There are some helpful educational tools available online which provide photos to demonstrate the wide range of normal vulval appearances [8].

Another cause for concern is if there is a disparity in the size of the labia. This is a common, temporary occurrence and requires reassurance that the two sides of the vulval will balance out, the larger sized labia having reached its adult size and the smaller side still growing. It would be advisable to wait until the girl is closer to adulthood and full development of the vulva before any surgical intervention could be considered. In many health systems this is only available in the private sector. If surgical labial reduction is considered, then the practitioner should be mindful of any safe-guarding concerns or any overlap with female genital mutilation (FGM) [9].

# CONGENITAL GYNAECOLOGICAL ANOMALIES

Uterine and vaginal congenital abnormalities are rare (<5% of the general female population) and are usually incidental findings at ultrasound for another clinical reason. They are usually asymptomatic (complete uterine didelphys/double uterus can sometimes present with menorrhagia) and typically become clinically relevant in relation to fertility and pregnancy [10].

## Imperforate hymen and hymenal septae

Imperforate hymen is rare (incidence 0.05–0.1%), however, despite the rarity of the condition it is easily diagnosed on history and examination, with classic clinical sign of a bulging and blue-tinged swelling in the vagina preceded by amenorrhoea despite the presence of secondary sexual characteristics (breast development, pubic and axillary hair) and cyclical abdominal pain, occasionally with urinary retention. Prompt surgical management in the form of excision or cruciate incision of the hymen is required to prevent long-term sequelae such as infections in the upper part of the female genital tract leading to sub-fertility [11].

Hymenal septae are more common, mainly vertical septae, and present in adolescence usually with difficulty with tampon use. Tampon use has increased in popularity with younger girls prior to becoming sexually active due to the small tampons available and the convenience associated with tampon use especially for sport and other activities. Typically, on history, the girls are able to insert the tampon, to one side of the septum, and then struggle to remove the tampon when it is enlarged due to absorption of menstrual fluid. This is when they see the septum. Often it is difficult to visualise the septum if a clinician is not experienced at this kind of examination, hence it is important to believe what the girl describes as having seen and then if required escalate/refer to secondary care to confirm and then manage the septum with a simple surgical division of the septum usually with diathermy.

## BREAST DISORDERS IN ADOLESCENCE

Breast awareness is a key part of overall awareness of health and lifestyle among adult women as well as adolescents. While breast awareness is encouraged and is now very much a part of the conscience of society, there are of course undue concerns caused by lack of information and understanding especially among very young women and teenage girls. There are many benign problems seen in young children and teenagers and we can address them in the following sub-groups.

## CONGENITAL/DEVELOPMENTAL ABNORMALITIES

Congenital anomalies can appear in the neonatal period in the form of residual breast buds which almost always settle once the baby is a few months old and this can affect both male and female babies. Other commonly found problems are super-numerary nipples (Polythelia) and super-numerary breast buds (Polymastia). Accessory breast tissue is most commonly seen within the axillae and can cause cyclical pain. None of these need any further investigations or intervention.

Breast hypoplasia is failure of one or both (rarely) breasts to develop fully and this is indeed a cause for concern especially as young girls attain menarche and thelarche. This could also be complicated by a rare congenital abnormality: Poland's syndrome which is absent or hypoplasia of pectoralis major muscle and varying degrees of syndactyly and is extremely rare and usually unilateral and partial in nature. Awareness of these conditions is extremely important for early diagnosis, reassurance and of course any treatment as required.

Tuberous breast is a developmental abnormality usually seen unilaterally but can also be bilateral. The manifestation of tuberous breasts can be very early at the time of puberty and while the advice is to wait for a few years until the patient has reached adulthood, it is important to acknowledge that tuberous breast in its severe form is not a self-correcting developmental abnormality and will require definitive surgical treatment if the patient so wishes. Cosmetic surgery is ideally not recommended in children and adolescents (under the age of 18 years) and the recommendation is to wait until the breast development and physical growth is complete before embarking on any corrective surgery. During this period, it would be helpful for the youngsters to be offered a prosthesis to correct asymmetry in clothing. The corrective surgery may require more than one procedure to correct the tuberous deformity and to attain symmetry of size and contour with the other breast and may also require corrective surgery to the other breast.

These abnormalities can cause significant mental and emotional distress in adolescents affecting their confidence, body image and ability to form relationships. It is important for clinicians to acknowledge, explain the underlying condition, re-assure and offer all options of treatment.

# ABERRATIONS OF NORMAL DEVELOPMENT AND INVOLUTION

Aberrations of normal process of breast development in adolescents is directly related to the breast development which is both stromal and lobular and can lead to juvenile hypertrophy, asymmetry or other developmental problems which are mostly cosmetic.

The most common findings of aberrations of normal development and involution (ANDI) are simple fibroadenomata in young women. These are benign, mobile lumps (breast mouse) and can be solitary or multiple and uni- or bilateral. Rapid growth of these fibroadneomata is rare outside adolescence and in this particular group is known as 'juvenile fibroadenomata' which can reach sizes of >5 cm (giant fibroadenoma).

Management of fibroadenoma in adolescents requires clinical examination and an ultrasound scan and core biopsies are not usually performed under 25 years of age. Excision of fibroadenoma is only recommended when it significantly increases in size over a short period of time, reaches >4 cm in size, or significantly distorts the breast profile especially in young girls with developing breasts. Surgical excision is usually a preferred option as this group of patients are too young for excision with vacuum-assisted mammotome under 'local anaesthetic'.

The other pathology which can present as a lump or nipple discharge (usually single duct and blood stained) can be intraduct papilloma in young women which can be single or multiple. Again, these are benign lumps and may require biopsy to prove that and in the instance of single duct clear discharge, a simple method of using urine dipstick test to look for occult blood is extremely helpful. Nipple discharge cytology is not going to be sufficiently useful to enable accurate diagnosis and treatment planning [12].

## Mastalgia

Mastalgia can be a common reason for referral to 'Specialist Breast Clinics' and can impact the patient significantly both physically and mentally. Cyclical mastalgia is almost always of hormonal aetiology and use of contraceptive pill can act as an exacerbating factor. Management of mastalgia involves assessment with history and examination in young adolescents and any radiological investigation is dependent on the clinical findings and is not recommended for mastalgia only.

Management of mastalgia includes significant reassurance, simple analgesia, cessation of smoking and decreasing caffeine intake. In young women with evolving and changing breast shape, size and contour, a well-fitting supportive bra and gentle stretching exercises are known to help the symptoms. Oil of evening primrose is recommended but does not have sufficient evidence to show benefit in any of the randomised crossover trials [13].

Breast infections are extremely rare in non-lactational young women except in smokers and clinical examination and breast imaging in the form of ultrasound scans are recommended before treatment with antibiotics and serial aspirations as required.

## Gynaecomastia

The most common condition affecting the male breast and involves hyperplasia of the stromal and ductal tissue of the male breast. It has to be differentiated from pseudo-gynaecomastia which is excessive adipose tissue with no increase in stromal or ductal tissue.

Causes of gynaecomastia in adults and young boys can be physiological/hormonal or drug induced (medicinal and recreational drugs). Biochemical assessment of prolactin, alpha-fetoprotein (AFP), beta-human gonadotropin (β-hCG) and total testosterone is only recommended in rapid growth and other associated features of endocrine abnormality and input from a paediatrician is not only recommended but absolutely essential in establishing diagnosis of underlying conditions. Routine imaging ± core biopsy is not essential for diagnosis of gynaecomastia in young adolescents.

Other causes of increased oestrogen secretion may need to be ruled out (for example, testicular tumours). Underlying endocrine abnormalities or chromosomal abnormalities leading to reduced production of androgens (e.g. Klinefelter's syndrome/hypogonadism/ hyperprolactinaemia/hypopituitarism, etc.) may need to be ruled out. Recreational drugs such as cannabis and heroin and body building drugs such as anabolic steroids are also known to be associated with causation of gynaecomastia.

Once the diagnosis has been established and underlying causes ruled out and gynaecomastia is confirmed as idiopathic, treatment involves reassurance, explanation of the condition and withdrawal of any medications or causative agents. While there are some drugs such as tamoxifen and danazole recommended for treatment of gynaecomastia, these are based on small non-randomised trials and do not include associated long-term risks or outcomes [14].

Surgery would be the definitive treatment option for moderate to severe gynaecomastia and will require excision of breast tissue ± liposuction ± reduction of excess redundant skin.

## CONCLUSION

Paediatricians have a vital role in diagnosing and managing many of the complex endocrine, genetic and congenital problems associated with physical and pubertal development. With children attaining puberty earlier, parents increasingly rely on their paediatricians for their expertise. An understanding of gynaecological and breast issues in children is vital in understanding whether reassurance is what the family needs, or if a referral to a specialist is necessary.

## REFERENCES

1.  Larcher V, Hutchinson A. How should paediatricians assess Gillick competence. Arch Dis Childhood 2010.
2.  Al-bedaery R, Brown H. Common adolescent and paediatric gynaecological referrals and the development of a targeted patient information leaflet. BJOG: Int J Obstet Gynaecol 2013; 346.
3.  Zannoni L, Giorgi M, Spagnolo E, et al. Dysmenorhea, absenteeism from school and symptoms suspicious of endometriosis in adolescents. J Pediatr Adolesc Gynaecol 2014; 258–265.
4.  BritsPAG: Guideline for the management of Heavy Menstrual Bleeding (HMB) in adolescents. www. BritsPag.org.uk
5.  Szydlarska D, Machaj M, Jakimiuk A. History of discovery of polycystic ovary syndrome. Advances in Clinical and Experimental Medicine. Poland: Wroclaw University of Medicine, 2017. Available from https://doi.org/10.17219/acem/61987 (Last accessed 23rd January 2023).
6.  Capozzi A, Scambia G, Lello S. Polycystic ovary syndrome (PCOS) and adolescence: How can we manage it? Eur J Obstet Gynecol Reprod Biol. Ireland: Elsevier Ireland Ltd., 2020. Available from https://doi.org/10.1016/j.ejogrb.2020.04.024 (Last accessed 23rd January 2023).
7.  BPJ. UK Medical Eligibility Criteria for Contraceptive Use (UKMEC). 2019. Available from https://bpac. org.nz/magazine/2008/april/docs/bpj12_ukmec_pages_28-29.pdf (Last accessed 23rd January 2023).

8.   Women's Health Victoria. The Labia Library. Women's Health Victoria. Melbourne. (2013). Available from http://www.labialibrary.org.au/ (Last accessed 23rd January 2023).

9.   Royal College of Obstetricians and Gynaecologists. Green Top Guideline 53: Female Genital Mutilation and Its Management. RCOG Green-top Guideline 2015; 53:1–26.

10.  Nahum GG. Uterine anomalies. How common are they and what it their distribution amongst subtypes. J Reprod Med 1998.

11.  Lee KH, Hong JS, Jung HJ, et al. Imperforate hymen: a comprehensive systematic review. J Clin Med 2019; 8:56.

12.  Kalu ON, Chow C, Wheeler A, Kong C, Wapnir I. The diagnostic value of nipple discharge cytology: breast imaging complements predictive value of nipple discharge cytology. J Surg Oncol 2012; 106:381–385.

13.  Blommers J, de Lange-De Klerk ES, Kuik DJ, Bezemer PD, Meijer S. Evening primrose oil and fish oil for severe chronic mastalgia: a randomized, double-blind, controlled trial. Am J Obstet Gynecol 2002; 187:1389–1394.

14.  Daniels IR, Layer GT. Gynaecomastia. Eur J Surg 2001; 167:885–892.

# Chapter 4

# Prenatal screening and diagnosis of genetic defects

*Tara Giacchino, Ranjit Akolekar*

## INTRODUCTION

Prenatal screening and diagnoses have rapidly evolved over the past few decades in parallel with advances in prenatal ultrasound techniques and improvements in genetic investigations. The aim of prenatal diagnosis is to provide women and their families with accurate information about their pregnancy regarding the genetic health so that they can make appropriate management plans based on these results. Depending on the nature of the genetic diagnosis, the management options available to a family and their clinical team include accurate results that can allow for close antenatal monitoring, specialist consultations with fetal medicine and genetics team, planning and preparation for optimal timing, mode and place of birth and need for specialist neonatal care. Also in some pregnancies, the option of considering a termination of pregnancy if the genetic defect is associated with substantial risk of perinatal death or severe handicap; the latter is subject to medical and legal guidelines that vary considerably among different countries. The knowledge of accurate prenatal diagnosis allows not just for effective management of the current pregnancy but provides information that can help in determining recurrence risks and management of future pregnancies.

## CHROMOSOMAL AND GENETIC ABNORMALITIES

Chromosomal and genetic abnormalities can be broadly divided into those that are numerical chromosomal abnormalities such as aneuploidies (e.g. trisomy or monosomy), those associated with loss or gain of genetic material such as deletions or duplications and those associated with change in a nucleotide base change such as DNA mutations. Genetic abnormalities can also be classified as those that are sporadic occurrences, i.e. that occur in a de novo fashion or those that are inherited from parents. Common examples of sporadic occurrences of genetic defects include primary trisomy or monosomy and

**Tara Giacchino** MD MRCOG MCh, Medway Fetal and Maternal Medicine Centre, Medway NHS Foundation Trust, Kent, UK
Email: tara.giacchino@nhs.net.

**Ranjit Akolekar** MBBS MD MRCOG, Medway Fetal and Maternal Medicine Centre, Medway NHS Foundation Trust and Institute of Medical Sciences, Canterbury Christ Church University, Rowan William's Court, Kent, UK
Email: ranjit.akolekar@nhs.net

**Table 4.1  Common types of chromosomal/genetic defects**

| Defect | Explanation | Examples |
|---|---|---|
| *De novo or sporadic defects* | | |
| Primary trisomy | Whole additional chromosome | Down's, Edward's and Patau's syndrome |
| Primary monosomy | Missing entire chromosome | Turner's syndrome |
| Triploidy | Whole extra set of chromosomes | Digynic or Diandric triploidy |
| Deletion or duplication | Part of a chromosome missing or duplicated | DiGeorge, Cri Du Chat and William's syndrome |
| Single gene mutation | DNA mutation in a single gene | Cornelia De Lange's syndrome |
| Chromosome re-arrangements | Isochromosome, marker chromosomes | Pallister–Killian's syndrome |
| *Inherited defects* | | |
| Secondary trisomy | Partial additional chromosome | Unbalanced translocation |
| Secondary monosomy | Partial missing chromosome | Unbalanced translocation |
| Deletion or duplication | Part of a chromosome missing or duplicated (as above) | Unbalanced translocation (as above) |
| *Single gene defects* | | |
| Autosomal dominant | Only one abnormal copy required for defect to express | Huntington's chorea |
| Autosomal recessive | Both copies abnormal for defect to express | Cystic fibrosis |
| Sex-linked | Defect on X-chromosome in 23rd pair | Duchenne muscular dystrophy |

deletions or duplications of parts of chromosomes whereas those that are inherited from parents include secondary trisomy or monosomy such as those inherited from parents carrying balanced chromosomal translocations when they become unbalanced and single gene disorders, i.e. DNA mutations those that are inherited from parents in a Mendelian fashion (e.g. recessive or dominant genetic defects, either autosomal or sex-linked) [1,2] (**Table 4.1**).

# PRENATAL SCREENING FOR CHROMOSOMAL/GENETIC DEFECTS

## Maternal risk factor-based screening

The most important risk factor associated with chromosomal abnormalities such as trisomy is maternal age. There is considerable evidence suggesting that the risk for fetal trisomies 13, 18 and 21, increases with maternal age. For example, the maternal age-related risk for trisomy-21, -18 and -13 at 12 weeks for a maternal age of 20 years is about

1 in 1,000, 1 in 2,500 and 1 in 8,000 whereas the same risks for the same gestation for a maternal age of 35 years is 1 in 250, 1 in 600 and 1 in 1,800 [3–5]. In contrast, the risk for other chromosomal abnormalities such as Turner's syndrome and 'triploidy' is unrelated to maternal age; the prevalence of these defects at 12 weeks is about 1 in 1,500 and 1 in 2,000. Maternal age was the method of screening in the 1970s and women over the age of 35 years, which constituted about 5% of the population at the time, were defined as screen positive and were offered further diagnostic testing for trisomy-21 with a detection rate (DR) of 30% [3–5].

## Serum-based screening

In the late 1980s and early 1990s, several studies demonstrated that in pregnancies with fetal trisomy-21 there are altered maternal serum concentrations of various biochemical markers, including increased free β-human chorionic gonadotropic (hCG) and inhibin A and decreased alpha-feto protein (AFP) and unconjugated oestriol 3 (uE3) [6–11]. These biochemical changes were combined with maternal age to develop the double test (hCG and AFP), triple test (hCG, AFP, and uE3) and the quadruple test (hCG, inhibin A, AFP, and uE3). Screening by this approach was superior to that of maternal age alone with DR of 50–70% at FPR of 5% [12]. However, these serum screening tests, i.e. triple, and quadruple tests were offered in the second trimester of pregnancy. As the advances occurred in fetal medicine, screening moved to the first trimester and it was realised that in pregnancies with fetal trisomies, there were significant alterations in concentrations of serum pregnancy associated plasma protein-A (PAPP-A) and free β-hCG in the first trimester of pregnancy [13,14]. The DR of trisomy-21 by first trimester biochemical markers was 60% for a false positive rate (FPR) of 5% [3].

## Ultrasound-based screening

### First trimester

An important milestone in prenatal screening was brought about by the introduction of ultrasound measurement of nuchal translucency (NT) at the first trimester 11–14-week scan. The seminal publication of the association of increased fetal NT thickness in pregnancies with trisomy-21 in 1992 and in the subsequent years demonstrated that a high proportion of affected pregnancies can be identified by ultrasound assessment of the fetus and measurement of fetal NT in first trimester [15–17]. For a FPR of 5%, screening by fetal NT thickness alone identifies about 75–80% of affected pregnancies. In addition to fetal NT thickness, other sensitive ultrasound markers of fetal trisomies at 11–13 weeks' scan include absence of fetal nasal bone, increased impedance to flow in fetal ductus venosus and tricuspid regurgitation, which are observed in about 60, 65, and 55% of pregnancies with trisomy-21, respectively [3,18–20].

### Second trimester

A detailed ultrasound scan carried out in the second trimester around 20 weeks allows for examination of fetal anatomy and genetic markers associated with fetal chromosomal and genetic defects. For example, trisomy-21 is associated with ventriculomegaly, nasal hypoplasia, nuchal oedema, cardiac defects, duodenal atresia and echogenic bowel, mild hydronephrosis, shortening of the femur and humerus. Similarly, trisomy-13 or -18 can be associated with brain abnormalities, facial cleft, micrognathia, nuchal oedema, heart defects, diaphragmatic hernia, exomphalos, single umbilical artery, renal defects, echogenic bowel, myelomeningocele, growth restriction and shortening of the limbs. The likelihood of association with fetal trisomy-21, given the presence of these markers was reported in a recent meta-analysis [21] (**Table 4.2**).

## Combined screening

In the 1990s, aneuploidy screening shifted to the first trimester with the 'Combined' test which uses ultrasound measurement of fetal NT together with maternal serum concentration of the placental proteins, free β-hCG and PAPP-A [3,15–17]. This combined test has a DR of 90% with FPR of 5% [3,17]. When combined screening is carried out with a combination of maternal age, fetal NT thickness, maternal serum free β-hCG and PAPP-A along with the additional ultrasound markers such as nasal bone, tricuspid valve and ductus venosus assessment, the DR can be improved to 96% for a FPR of 3% [22–24] (**Table 4.3**). The use of these additional ultrasound markers can be used in universal screening for all pregnancies but can also be used in a contingent screening policy whereby universal

| Table 4.2   Likelihood ratios of ultrasound markers with fetal trisomy-21 [21] | | | |
|---|---|---|---|
| Marker | Positive LR | Negative LR | LR isolated marker |
| Intra-cardiac echogenic focus | 5.85 | 0.80 | 0.95 |
| Ventriculomegaly | 25.78 | 0.94 | 3.57 |
| Increased nuchal fold | 19.18 | 0.80 | 3.12 |
| Echogenic bowel | 11.44 | 0.90 | 1.65 |
| Mild hydronephrosis | 7.77 | 0.92 | 1.10 |
| Short humerus | 4.81 | 0.74 | 0.78 |
| Short femur | 3.72 | 0.80 | 0.61 |
| Aberrant right subclavian artery | 21.48 | 0.71 | 3.94 |
| Absent or hypoplastic nasal bone | 23.26 | 0.46 | 6.58 |
| (LR, likelihood ratio) | | | |

| Table 4.3. Performance of different methods of screening for trisomy-21 [3] | | |
|---|---|---|
| Method of screening | DR (%) | FPR (%) |
| Maternal age | 30 | 5 |
| Maternal age + fetal NT | 75–80 | 5 |
| Maternal age + fetal NT + serum free β-hCG and PAPP-A (combined screening) | 85–95 | 5 |
| Combined screening + nasal bone + tricuspid flow + ductus venosus flow | 93–96 | 2.5 |
| (DR, detection rate; FPR, false positive rate; hCG, human chorionic gonadotropin; NT, nuchal translucency; PAPP-A, pregnancy-associated plasma protein) | | |

screening is carried out using maternal age, fetal NT and serum biochemistry and those with a high-risk result of <1 in 50 can be offered further invasive testing, those with a low risk of <1:1,000 are reassured and those in the intermediate risk group of 1 in 51 to 1 in 1,000 are offered further specialist ultrasound assessment with these ultrasound markers [3,25].

## DNA-based screening

In the late 1990s, it was discovered that free fetal DNA can be identified in maternal blood [26,27]. This cell-free (cf)-DNA in maternal plasma is a mixture of DNA fragments belonging to both the mother and fetus. The proportion of fetal to total cfDNA, referred to as fetal fraction is about 10% [28]. Recent advances in genetic technologies such as digital polymerase chain reaction (PCR), massively parallel sequencing and single nucleotide polymorphism (SNP) based methods have made it feasible to quantify these small increases in fetal cfDNA amount in trisomic pregnancies [29–31]. There have been several studies published in the last decade which demonstrate effectiveness of screening for fetal trisomies using the cfDNA. A recent meta-analysis demonstrated that in screening for trisomy-21, the weighted pooled DR and FPR were 99.7% and 0.04%, respectively. Similarly, for trisomy-13 and -18, the DR were 99.0% and 97.9%, respectively with corresponding FPR of 0.04% and 0.04%, respectively [32,33].

# PRENATAL DIAGNOSIS FOR CHROMOSOMAL/GENETIC DEFECTS

## Invasive prenatal diagnostic tests

Amniocentesis and chorionic villus sampling (CVS) are commonly performed procedures for invasive prenatal diagnosis. Women who are deemed to be at an increased risk for chromosomal abnormalities or those with a family history of an affected pregnancy are offered these diagnostic tests for further investigation. The aim is to obtain fetal DNA either from the placental (CVS) or the amniotic fluid (amniocentesis). These procedures are relatively safe with recent cohort studies and systemic reviews demonstrating that in pregnancies undergoing these invasive procedures, the procedure-related risk of pregnancy loss of about 0.3–0.5% [34,35]. CVS is generally preferred as it allows prenatal diagnosis at an earlier gestation and therefore provides reassurance if the results are normal. Furthermore, if the results are abnormal, CVS facilitates decision making at an earlier gestation, compared to amniocentesis, as CVS can be carried out at or after 11 weeks' gestation whilst amniocentesis can be carried out at or after 15 weeks' gestation.

## Laboratory genetic tests

Once genetic material is obtained for further laboratory investigation following a CVS or an amniocentesis, the tests available depend on the clinical indication for prenatal diagnosis. The common laboratory investigations include quantitative fluorescence polymerase chain reaction (QF-PCR), fluorescent in-situ hybridisation (FISH), karyotyping and comparative genomic hybridisation (CGH) array or SNP array, whole exome sequencing (WES) and molecular genetic testing for DNA mutations.

QF-PCR amplifies chromosome-specific DNA sequences or short tandem repeats and uses fluorescent primers to identify and quantify the amplified sequences as 'peak areas' on automated machines. Normal heterozygous individuals demonstrate two peak areas for each chromosome while those with trisomies will show an extra peak or an imbalanced peak ratio [36]. QF-PCR also provides rapid result within 3 days and can only be used to detect the common aneuploidies (T21, T13, and T18), sex chromosome abnormalities and triploidies.

FISH involves preparing fluorescent-labelled 'probes' or short sequences of single-stranded DNA that match up with the gene mutation being investigated for and bridges the gap between cytogenetics and molecular DNA testing. FISH can be done if early diagnosis is needed as the result is known in 24 hours; however, a positive result obtained by FISH needs to be reconfirmed by micro-array or karyotype [37,38]. FISH is advantageous as it detects subtle changes in chromosomes like duplications or deletions and can be done to interphase nuclei of non-mitotic cells. Therefore, the long process of cell culture is not needed, making it an ideal test in pre-implantation genetic diagnosis as it is quick [39]. Both FISH and QF-PCR need confirmation from the final karyotype; QF-PCR is often preferred over FISH as it requires few cells, is cheaper and as an automated machine is used, many samples can run concurrently and quickly.

Fetal karyotype with G-banding is the gold standard cytogenetic test for prenatal diagnosis of chromosomal abnormalities or aneuploidy and involves looking at the number as well as the structure or characteristic banding pattern of the 23 chromosome pairs. G-banding involves the use of Giemsa staining to divide a chromosome into regions, bands and sub-bands to detect abnormalities or re-arrangements like deletions, translocations, insertions or inversions. The sensitivity and specificity of this testing is nearly 99%, except for cases where confined placental mosaicism is present, and the fetal DNA sample was obtained by CVS [40].

Micro-array-based comparative genomic hybridisation (array CGH) directly compares DNA from two genomes, i.e. the patient and the control or reference which are uniquely fluorescently labelled and co-hybridised on a solid microscope slide with hundreds or thousands of immobilised DNA fragments or 'targets'. The advantage of this test with several overlapping targets, over FISH or other molecular cytogenetic tests is the detection of simultaneous DNA mutations at different loci in a given genome including deletions, duplications, or copy number imbalances [41,42]. In comparison, the highest resolution for standard karyotyping by G-banding is 3 Mb, for FISH is 1–2 Mb with the best resolution of 1 Kb obtained by aCGH. It can be considered as reliable as conventional karyotyping at diagnosing aneuploidy and unbalanced mutations. The limitations of chromosomal microarray include inability to detect single nucleotide mutations, abnormalities associated with balanced translocations, mosaicism and triploidy [43,44]. This led to another type of test known as SNPs array which involves the analysis of small segments of DNA affecting one nucleotide base which can detect small abnormalities including triploidy [45].

*Whole exome sequencing (WES)* has been introduced to better prenatal diagnosis when structural abnormalities have been confirmed on ultrasound or if there is a family history of consanguinity or similar fetal abnormalities without a genetic diagnosis. WES detects aberrations in the protein coding region of the genome and any changes to the norm are known as variants which can be categorised as pathogenic, likely pathogenic, benign, likely benign or of unknown significance. The improved diagnostic yield ranges from 10 to 50% and is case dependant and highly dependent on the indication for WES [46].

# CONCLUSION

- Common genetic and chromosomal defects include aneuploidies, chromosomal or genetic deletions or duplications, chromosome re-arrangements and single nucleotide changes.
- Chromosomal and genetic abnormalities can either occur in a sporadic or de novo fashion with no significant implications for future pregnancies or could be inherited from parents who are carriers of balanced chromosome re-arrangements or single gene disorders.
- The management of pregnancies at high-risk of chromosomal or genetic defects should be undertaken with specialists in fetal medicine and clinical genetics.
- The current method of prenatal screening for fetal trisomies is combined screening in the first trimester which estimates an individual patient-specific risk based on maternal age, fetal NT thickness and serum biochemistry (free $\beta$-hCG and PAPP-A). Additional ultrasound markers in the first trimester such as nasal bone, tricuspid and ductus venosus flow, improve DR and reduce FPR.
- cfDNA-based screening for fetal trisomies is highly accurate and identifies >99% of affected pregnancies at a low FPR of <0.1%.
- Common tests to obtain samples for prenatal diagnosis include CVS and amniocentesis, which can be carried out after 11 and 15 weeks, respectively.
- QF-PCR and FISH can be used for rapid prenatal diagnosis of aneuploidies with results available in 24–48 hours.
- Chromosome re-arrangements including deletions and duplications can be effectively identified using G-banding karyotype and micro-array-based techniques such as CGH and SNP array. The micro-array-based techniques have a higher resolution and are better in detecting smaller genetic changes.

# REFERENCES

1. Homfray T. Genetic Conditions: Chromosomal and Single Gene Disorders and Non-invasive Prenatal Testing. Glob Libr Women's Med 2021.
2. Mckinlay Gardner RJ, Amor DJ. Gardner and Sutherland's Chromosome Abnormalities and Genetic Counseling, 5th edition. Oxford Monograph Med Genet 2018.
3. Nicolaides KH. Screening for fetal aneuploidies at 11 to 13 weeks. Prenat Diagn 2011; 31:7–15.
4. Snijders RJM, Sebire NJ, Cuckle H, Nicolaides KH. Maternal age and gestational age-specific risks for chromosomal defects. Fetal Diagn Ther 1995; 10:356–367.
5. Snijders RJM, Sundberg K, Holzgreve W, Henry G, Nicolaides KH. Maternal age and gestation-specific risk for trisomy 21. Ultrasound Obstet Gynecol 1999; 13:167–170.
6. Merkatz IR, Nitowsky HM, Macri JN, Johnson WE. An association between low maternal serum alpha-fetoprotein and fetal chromosomal abnormalities. Am J Obstet Gynecol 1984; 148:886–894.
7. Aitken DA, Wallace EM, Crossley JA, et al. Dimeric inhibin A as a marker for Down's syndrome in early pregnancy. N Engl J Med 1996; 334:1231–1236.
8. Brambati B, Macintosh MCM, Teisner B, et al. Low maternal serum level of pregnancy associated plasma protein (PAPP-A) in the first trimester in association with abnormal fetal karyotype. BJOG 1993; 100:324–326.
9. Canick J, Knight GJ, Palomaki GE, et al. Low second trimester maternal serum unconjugated oestriol in pregnancies with Down's syndrome. BJOG 1988; 95:330–333.
10. Macri JN, Kasturi RV, Krantz DA, et al. Maternal serum Down syndrome screening: free beta protein is a more effective marker than human chorionic gonadotrophin. Am J Obstet Gynecol 1990; 163:1248–1253.

11. Van Lith JM, Pratt JJ, Beekhuis JR, Mantingh A. Second trimester maternal serum immuno-reactive inhibin as a marker for fetal Down's syndrome. Prenat Diagn 1993; 12:801–806.
12. Cuckle H, Benn P, Wright D. Down syndrome screening in the first and/or second trimester: model predicted performance using meta-analysis parameters. Semin Perinatol 2005; 29:252–257.
13. Spencer K, Tul N, Nicolaides KH. Maternal serum free beta hCG and PAPP-A in fetal sex chromsome defects in the first trimester. Prenat Diagn 2000; 20:390–394.
14. Kagan KO, Wright D, Spencer K, Molina FS, Nicolaides KH. First trimester screening for trisomy 21 by free beta-human chorionic gonadotropin and pregnancy-associated plasma protein-A: impact of maternal and pregnancy characteristics. Ultrasound Obstet Gynecol 2008; 31:493–502.
15. Nicolaides KH, Azar G, Byrne D, Mansur C, Marks K. Fetal nuchal translucency: ultrasound screening for chromosomal defects in first trimester of pregnancy. Br Med J 1992; 304:867–889.
16. Snijders RJ, Noble P, Sebire N, Souka A, Nicolaides KH. Fetal Medicine Foundation First Trimester Screening Group. UK multicentre project on assessment of risk of trisomy 21 by maternal age and fetal nuchal-translucency thickness at 10–14 weeks of gestation. Lancet 1998; 352:343–346.
17. Kagan KO, Wright D, Baker A, Sahota D, Nicolaides KH. Screening for trisomy 21 by maternal age, fetal nuchal translucency thickness, free beta-human chorionic gonadotropin and pregnancy associated plasma protein-A. Ultrasound Obstet Gynecol 2008; 31:618–624.
18. Matias A, Gomes C, Flack N, Montenegro N, Nicolaides KH. Screening for chromosomal abnormalities at 10–14 weeks: the role of ductus venosus blood flow. Ultrasound Obstet Gynecol 1998; 12:380–384.
19. Cicero S, Curcio P, Papageorghiou A, Sonek J, Nicolaides KH. Absence of nasal bone in fetuses with Trisomy 21 at 11–14 weeks of gestation: an observational study. Lancet 2001; 358:1665–1667.
20. Huggon IC, DeFigueiredo DB, Allan LD. Tricuspid regurgitation in the diagnosis of chromosomal anomalies in the fetus at 11–14 weeks of gestation. Heart 2003; 89:1071–1073.
21. Agathokleous M, Chaveeva P, Poon LC, Kosinski P, Nicolaides KH. Meta-analysis of second-trimester markers for trisomy 21. Ultrasound Obstet Gynecol. 2013; 41:247–261.
22. Kagan KO, Cicero S, Staboulidou I, Wright D, Nicolaides KH. Fetal nasal bone in screening for trisomies 21, 18 and 13 and Turner syndrome at 11–13 weeks of gestation. Ultrasound Obstet Gynecol 2009; 33:259–264.
23. Kagan KO, Valencia C, Livanos P, Wright D, Nicolaides KH. Tricuspid regurgitation in screening for trisomies 21, 18 and 13 and Turner syndrome at $11^{+0}–13^{+6}$ weeks of gestation. Ultrasound Obstet Gynecol 2009; 33:18–22.
24. Maiz N, Valencia C, Kagan KO, Wright D, Nicolaides KH. Ductus venosus Doppler in screening for trisomies 21, 18 and 13 and Turner syndrome at 11–13 weeks of gestation. Ultrasound Obstet Gynecol 2009; 33:512–517.
25. Kagan KO, Staboulidou I, Cruz J, Wright D, Nicolaides KH. Two-stage first-trimester screening for trisomy 21 by ultrasound assessment and biochemical testing. Ultrasound Obstet Gynecol 2010; 36:524–547.
26. Lo YM, Corbetta N, Chamberlain PF, et al. Presence of fetal DNA in maternal plasma and serum. Lancet 1997; 350:485–487.
27. Lo YM, Tein MS, Lau TK, et al. Quantitative analysis of fetal DNA in maternal plasma and serum: implications for noninvasive prenatal diagnosis. Am J Hum Genet 1998; 62:768–775.
28. Ashoor G, Syngelaki A, Poon LC, Rezende JC, Nicolaides KH. Fetal fraction in maternal plasma cell-free DNA at 11-13 weeks' gestation: relation to maternal and fetal characteristics. Ultrasound Obstet Gynecol 2013; 41:26–32.
29. Palomaki GE, Kloza EM, Lambert-Messerlian GM, et al. DNA sequencing of maternal plasma to detect Down syndrome: An international clinical validation study. Genet Med 2011; 13:913–920.
30. Pergament E, Cuckle H, Zimmermann B, et al. Single-nucleotide polymorphism-based noninvasive prenatal screening in a high-risk and low-risk cohort. Obstet Gynecol 2014; 124:210–218.
31. Song Y, Liu C, Qi H, et al. Noninvasive prenatal testing of fetal aneuploidies by massively parallel sequencing in a prospective Chinese population. Prenat Diagn 2013; 33:700–706.
32. Gil MM, Akolekar R, Quezada MS, Bregant B, Nicolaides KH. Analysis of cell-free DNA in maternal blood in screening for aneuploidies: meta-analysis. Fetal Diagn Ther 2014; 35:156–173.

33. Gil MM, Accurti V, Santacruz B, Plana MN, Nicolaides KH. Analysis of cell-free DNA in maternal blood in screening for aneuploidies: updated meta-analysis. Ultrasound Obstet Gynecol 2017; 50:302–314.

34. Beta J, Zhang W, Geris S, Kostiv V, Akolekar R. Procedure-related risk of miscarriage from chorionic villus and amniocentesis. Ultrasound in Obstet Gynaecol 2019; 54:452–457.

35. Akolekar R, Beta J, Picciarelli G, Ogilvie C, D'Antonio F. Procedure-related risk of miscarriage following amniocentesis and chorionic villus sampling: a systematic review and meta-analysis. Ultrasound Obstet Gynecol 2015; 45:16–26.

36. Adinolfi M, Pertl B, Sherlock J. Rapid detection of aneuploidies by microsatellite and the quantitative fluorescent polymerase chain reaction. Prenat Diagn 1997; 17:1299–1311.

37. Evans MI, Ebrahim SAD, Berry SM, et al. Fluorescent in situ hybridization utilization for high-risk prenatal diagnosis: a trade-off among speed, expense, and inherent limitations of chromosomes specific probes. Am J Obstet Gynecol 1994; 171:1055–1057.

38. Toutain J, Epiney M, Begorre M, et al. First-trimester prenatal diagnosis performed on pregnant women with fetal ultrasound abnormalities: the reliability of interphase fluorescence in situ hybridization (FISH) on mesenchymal core for the mail aneuploidies. Eur J Obstet Gynecol Reprod Biol 2010; 21:293–301.

39. Verlinsky Y, Cieslak J, Freidine M, et al. Polar body diagnosis of common aneuploidies by FISH. J Assist Reprod Genet 1996; 13:157–162.

40. Jelin AC, Sagaser KG, Wilkins-Haug L. Prenatal Genetic Testing Options. Pediatric Clin North Am 2019; 66:281–293.

41. Bejjani BA, Shaffer LG. Application of array-based comparative genomic hybridization to clinical diagnostics. J Mol Diagn 2006; 8:528–533.

42. Kashork CD, Theisen A, Shaffer LG. Prenatal diagnosis using array CGH. Methods Mol Biol 2008; 444:59–69.

43. American College of Obstetricians and Gynecologists Committee on Genetics. Committee Opinion No. 581: The use of chromosomal microarray analysis in prenatal diagnosis. Obstet Gynecol 2013; 122:1374–1377.

44. Wapner RJ, Martin CL, Levy B, et al. Chromosomal microarray versus karyotyping for prenatal diagnosis. N Engl J Med 2012; 367:2175–2184.

45. Fox CE, Kilby MD. Prenatal diagnosis in the modern era. Obstet Gynaecol 2016; 18:213–219.

46. Richards S, Aziz N, Bale S, et al. Standards and guidelines for the interpretation of sequence variants: a joint consensus recommendation of the American College of Medical Genetics and Genomics and the Association for Molecular Pathology. Genet Med 2015; 17:405–424.

# Chapter 5

# Advances in neonatal care

*Jessica Burgess-Shannon, Deena-Shefali Patel, Cheryl Battersby*

## INTRODUCTION

Improvements in neonatal care over the past 30 years have seen a dramatic reduction in mortality [1]. Globally, neonatal deaths have fallen from 5 million in 1990 to 2.4 in 2019 [1]. However, the majority of childhood deaths still occurs within the neonatal period. Prematurity, perinatal asphyxia, infections and congenital anomalies are the most common causes [1]. While not every death is avoidable, effective preparation and delivery room management reduce mortality and morbidity. In this chapter we discuss four key areas of neonatal care from a global perspective, acknowledging that some may be more relevant to high income country settings: (i) Antenatal, delivery room stabilisation and resuscitation (ii) Respiratory management, in particular strategies to reduce bronchopulmonary dysplasia or chronic lung disease (iii) Family-integrated care (iv) Antenatal and postnatal screening. For each area, we highlight where practice has changed, where controversies or uncertainties remain and future directions.

## BIRTH AND RESUSCITATION

### Antenatal care

Neonatal outcomes are influenced by factors occurring long before birth. Focus has shifted towards actively managing modifiable prenatal exposures to provide newborns with the best possible start. This includes optimising maternal health through screening, treatment of pregnancy-related complications, and effectively managing preterm labour

**Jessica Burgess-Shannon** MBChB BSc (hons) MRCPCH and PG Cert, Neonatal Specialist Grid Trainee, Chelsea and Westminster Hospital, London, UK
Email: j.burgess-shannon@nhs.net

**Deena-Shefali Patel** MBBS PgCert Healthcare ethics and Law MD (Res) FRCPCH, Neonatal Consultant, Chelsea and Westminster Hospital, Honorary lecturer Imperial College London, London, UK
Email: deena-shefali.patel@nhs.net

**Cheryl Battersby** BMedSci BMBS PhD FRCPCH, Clinical Senior Lecturer in Neonatal Medicine, National Institute for Health and Care Research (NIHR) Clinician Scientist, Honorary Neonatal Consultant, Chelsea and Westminster Hospital, London, UK
Email: c.battersby@imperial.ac.uk

with tocolytics if appropriate, antibiotics for suspected infection/premature prolonged rupture of membranes (pPROM), along with provision of antenatal corticosteroids and magnesium sulphate [2–10]. Antenatal corticosteroids have been shown to reduce the risk of death, respiratory distress syndrome (RDS), as well as intra-ventricular haemorrhage (IVH), and magnesium sulphate to neuroprotection for preterm infants [11,12]. However, in recent years, the benefits and possible harms of antenatal corticosteroids were called into question, particularly in low-resource countries and in late preterm infants [13]. The WHO ACTION-I trial conducted in low-resource countries has resulted in new 2022 WHO recommendations including the overarching recommendation for administering antenatal corticosteroids to women with a high likelihood of preterm birth from 24 weeks to an upper limit of 34+0 weeks of gestation [14,15]. The caveat to this being the possible need for reorganisation of healthcare resources and systems, particularly in low- and middle-income countries (LMIC), to achieve effective implementation [15]. More research is needed to determine the optimum timing, dosing and gestational age groups who would confer most benefit from antenatal steroids [15]. There is evidence to support the transfer of high-risk pregnancies, including extremely preterm infants likely to deliver, before birth to a centre with the appropriate expertise in providing care to improve outcomes [16–18].

## Essential delivery room stabilisation

Most infants physiologically adapt to extra-uterine life without event, with evidence to suggest 70–80% of extremely preterm infants will establish breathing without intervention, and it is increasingly recognised that most preterm babies require support to transition rather than resuscitation [19]. Evidence-based interventions to support transition in preterm infants include deferred cord clamping (DCC), early continuous positive airway pressure (CPAP) support and effective thermoregulation [20–29].

Deferred cord clamping (DCC) reduces mortality, IVH, the need for blood transfusion and inotropic support for preterm infants and all major resuscitation groups support DCC for at least 1 minute in stable newborns [20–24]. More research is needed to determine the optimal duration of DCC, which may vary for different gestations. Greater provision of DCC may result from the use of bedside platforms providing the opportunity for simultaneous stabilisation and may have the additional benefit of proximity to parents if support is required [30–32].

Umbilical cord milking (UCM) has been explored as an alternative, particularly in the context of a baby that requires immediate resuscitation but is not actively supported by the current neonatal life support (NLS), European Resuscitation Council (ERC) and American Heart Association (AHA) for extremely preterm babies [21–23]. A recent systematic review highlighted a statistically significant increased risk of IVH with UCM compared to DCC for preterm infants [33]. While the included studies were heterogeneous in nature and affected by their own individual biases, the findings still warrant caution in the absence of further evidence.

Airway and ventilation strategy has changed over recent years as an understanding of the need to avoid mechanical ventilation and thus ventilator-associated lung injury has evolved. This extends to delivery room practice where there has been a move away from routine intubation and prophylactic surfactant administration in favour of stabilisation on CPAP. Use of CPAP results in reduced rates of chronic lung disease (CLD) and death compared to mechanical ventilation, and should be established early in the delivery room for spontaneously breathing preterm infants [21–27].

## Extreme preterm management

Resuscitation at the limits of viability is a matter of much debate across high-income countries (HIC) where improving survival rates and neuro-developmental outcomes have been shown [34–39]. In some countries, such as the UK, there has been a move away from decision-making on gestation alone, in favour of considering key prognostic factors in consultation with parents [35]. Others have opted for a uniformly active approach to infants born at the extremes of prematurity, such as Sweden where a recent study demonstrated 52% survival for infants born at 22 weeks, with 66% being unimpaired at 2.5-year follow-up [40].

We anticipate that the evolving experience of managing these infants will improve outcomes over time. Japan has some of the highest survival rates for extremely preterm infants globally. There the limit of viability changed from 24 to 22 weeks as early as 1991 in some centres [41–42]. Over time survival for 22-week infants receiving resuscitation increased in Japan from 35.0% in 2003–2007 compared to 46.1% in 2008–2012; and 60.7–72.9% over the same time periods for infants born at 23 weeks [43].

The highest burden of preterm birth is in low-to-middle income countries (LMIC), as it is the greatest disparity in outcomes [2,44]. The World Health Organization's 'Born Too Soon' report highlights a 50% chance of survival for infants born at 24 weeks in most HIC, while a comparative chance of survival is not seen until 34 weeks in LMIC settings [9]. Cost-effective interventions that improve outcomes in all settings, such as comprehensive antenatal care, thermoregulation, infection control and nutrition remain the immediate priority in tackling this inequality [2].

## Resuscitation

A minority of preterm and term infants require active resuscitation at birth, and it is essential that neonatal practitioners are trained to provide this. All major resuscitation guidelines are united in their approach of establishing an open airway, effectively aerating the lungs, and then progressing to chest compressions and drugs for the few who do not respond [21–24,45].

Supraglottic airway (SGA) devices, such as the laryngeal mask airway (LMA), facilitate airway support for neonatal care providers without comprehensive intubation skills. Studies from the low-resource setting comparing intermittent positive pressure ventilation (IPPV) via LMA and face mask have found improved short-term outcomes in the LMA group, with one study demonstrating shorter time to spontaneous breathing, and positive long-term outcomes with no differences in early mortality and hypoxic ischaemia encephalopathy (HIE) [46,47]. While the evidence base for LMAs largely derives from studies in LMIC, their relevance translates to all settings as we move towards a less invasive approach, further compounded by the potential impact of this on airway skills of clinicians [48–51]. The most recent Cochrane review concluded that using a LMA is not only more effective than face mask IPPV, but comparable with IPPV via endotracheal tube (ETT) intubation [52]. Unfortunately, at present, SGA devices have size limitations. ERC and NLS recommend use of the size 1.0 device in infants ≥34 weeks and ≥1,500–2,000 g, respectively [21,22]. In RCTs, LMAs have been used in infants as small as 1 kg [48]. The development of smaller equipment may increase their use further.

Other changes in equipment include the routine use of saturation probes to monitor and target oxygen administration along with recommendations for capnography to confirm ETT placement, in conjunction with clinical indicators [21–24]. ECG appears to provide faster and more accurate heart rate assessment in comparison to auscultation, palpation and pulse oximetry and may well become more commonplace in delivery room management over time [21–24,53,54].

Drugs of resuscitation are another area of debate. Theoretically, correcting acidosis with sodium bicarbonate optimises the physiological environment for myocardial and adrenaline function. This assumption largely derives from animal and in vitro models suggesting that acidosis debilitates adrenaline binding to target receptors, along with animal studies showing superiority of intravenous bases over respiratory stimulants in resuscitation situations [55–57]. Only one small clinical trial exists; the study randomised newborns requiring IPPV at five minutes to sodium bicarbonate or placebo and found no difference in death or abnormal neurological examination at discharge [58,59]. It is difficult to extrapolate these results primarily due to the differences in the groups and also only a proportion of both groups received chest compressions prior to drug administration. Concerns are further compounded by evidence that sodium bicarbonate creates a hyperosmolar load and increases carbon dioxide levels, paradoxically worsening acidosis, albeit this latter finding has not been replicated in resuscitation studies [60–62]. Neither the evidence to support nor refute the use of sodium bicarbonate is conclusive, thus there has been a move away from routine use but it should still be considered in prolonged resuscitation [21,22,24].

Supporting parents to be present at resuscitations is now generally advocated. Concerns regarding a negative impact on neonatal outcomes, staff performance and the psychological burden on parents have not been borne out in the available research, and it may indeed provide benefit [63–66].

## Future directions

There is much still to learn about optimal delivery room management. Interesting work into the optimal interface for CPAP is ongoing following a recent observational study highlighting apnoea as a possible sequelae to face mask application in preterm infants [67,68]. The role of delivery room surfactant is being revisited, in the era of less invasive management, with preliminary data on catheter administration (known as Minimally Invasive Surfactant Therapy, or MIST), LMA therapy and oropharyngeal installation beginning to evolve [69–71]. At present, the majority of delivery room ventilation for intubated infants is pressure-limited, with non-humidified gases. Given the concerns of damage to the preterm lung with even a short period of ventilation it will be interesting to see if delivery room volume targeted ventilation, and humidified gases have an impact on outcomes [72–74].

# STRATEGIES TO REDUCE CHRONIC LUNG DISEASE

Reducing morbidity and mortality from preterm respiratory conditions, namely RDS and CLD, is a key area of interest. CLD is associated with increased mortality along with long-lasting respiratory and neuro-developmental sequelae [74–81].

## Non-invasive support

Optimising respiratory status starts before birth with the provision of antenatal steroids and continues with the choice of early CPAP for spontaneously breathing infants [11,21–27].

The shift towards a less invasive approach is an entire movement. Techniques to facilitate surfactant administration via less invasive methods have evolved to provide the benefits of improved lung compliance while avoiding the disadvantages of mechanical ventilation. MIST, also known as Less Invasive Surfactant Administration (LISA), involves passing a thin catheter into the trachea for a short period and instilling surfactant while maintaining CPAP. At meta-analysis, MIST is associated with a reduction in death/CLD at 36 weeks, CLD among survivors and need for mechanical ventilation in comparison to conventional methods [82]. Recent reviews have concluded that the current evidence base supports MIST over techniques, such as 'InSurE', whereby infants are intubated with an ETT and subsequently extubated [25,26,83,84].

There is significant variation in practice regarding sedation for MIST and some clinicians elect to use no drugs at all. Sedative medication may improve the chance of success with a calm infant, and increase comfort. This must be balanced with the risk of respiratory depression that may necessitate intubation and ventilation [85,86]. The optimal timing of treatment requires further exploration, while the current evidence base supports MIST in the context of early rescue, the benefit of routine prophylaxis in the delivery room has not yet been fully evaluated but is practiced in some centres [84,86]. Operator experience is a further challenge especially if MIST is administered via direct laryngoscopy where there is no shared view. Video-laryngoscopy may overcome this barrier and support trainees to develop their skills [84].

While current guidelines advocate for CPAP as the first-line non-invasive approach for respiratory support, humidified high-flow nasal cannula (HHFNC) has been explored as an alternative [21–24,29–31]. HHFNC delivers substantial flow rates of humidified, blended air/oxygen through prongs inserted into the nose to reduce effort of breathing; this is likely to be achieved by providing an unmeasured positive end-expiratory pressure that reduces functional residual capacity, and reducing the physiological dead space. A 2016 Cochrane inclusive of four studies comparing CPAP to HHFNC concluded that efficacy was comparable after finding no difference in the primary outcome of death or CLD, although duration of support was increased in the HHFNC group [87]. The included studies however largely exclude the most preterm infants with the lowest inclusion gestation of any paper being 27 weeks [87]. More recent meta-analyses are limited by the same biases [88]. Results for HHFNC compared to CPAP following extubation appear similar, although the 2021 meta-analysis identified lower rates of treatment failure in favour of CPAP, with lower risks of nasal breakdown and pneumothorax in the HHFNC group [87,88]. The trepidation regarding HHFNC is whether it results in greater atelectasis; more research is needed to draw conclusions, particularly as the most preterm infants remain unrepresented in the available research.

## Gentle ventilation strategies

When ventilation is necessary, a protective strategy should be employed that aims to minimise injury [25–27]. Traditional conventional ventilation modes can either deliver a set pressure, or set volume, with the other parameter varying within specified limits to achieve the desired settings. At meta-analysis volume targeted ventilation (VTV) is consistently associated with improved outcomes compared to pressure-limited modes with reduced risk of death or CLD, pneumothorax, severe IVH, hypocarbia and shorter duration of mechanical ventilation [89,90].

In the environment in which resources are limited, even when ventilators are available, additional equipment may be needed to deliver the ventilation modes advocated for in HIC; VTV, for example, requires a flow sensor for accurate delivery. These factors must be considered when developing local guidelines and research in LMIC which supports understanding of optimal respiratory support in different settings [91–94].

## Oxygen control

Optimal target saturations for preterm infants have been the subject of much research with the balance of favour thought to fall on the side of targeting 91–95% due to reduced rates of mortality and NEC, compared to 85–89%, although risk of CLD and ROP increases [25–27,95]. Servo-controlled oxygen titration systems alter oxygen delivery based on saturations. The available evidence suggests this innovation results in increased time within target range compared to manual adjustment, however, the impact on morbidity and mortality is yet to be addressed [96–99].

## Postnatal steroids

Ongoing mechanical ventilation, though necessary for some infants, is damaging to the preterm lung and contributes to the pathogenesis of CLD. The anti-inflammatory properties of postnatal corticosteroids make them an attractive option for infants who remain ventilator dependent. The benefits and risks of postnatal steroids are clear but questions remain regarding optimal therapeutic agents, dosage, timing and delivery [100–103].

Multiple studies looking at dosing and timing have been undertaken; some like the low-dose dexamethasone DART trial showed promising results but a significant under recruitment provided data that cannot be confidently interpreted [104,105]. The more recent PREMILOC study has renewed interest in the use of early low-dose hydrocortisone after finding reduced rates of CLD with no increased risk of gastrointestinal (GI) perforation or impact on neuro-developmental outcomes at 2-year follow-up [106,112]. There were however higher rates of sepsis in the 24–25 weeks subgroup and again long-term data are lacking [111].

Multiple meta-analyses have followed and in essence have concluded that it is likely that systemic steroids used after the first week of life have a beneficial effect on duration of mechanical ventilation, CLD and mortality, however, due to the heterogeneity of included studies and a lack of long-term data the question of neuro-developmental impact has been harder to answer [101,106,107]. A detrimental effect cannot be ruled out, neither can an assumption that improved respiratory outcomes will confer neuro-developmental benefit. Clinicians remain divided in their approach to the ventilator-dependent infant, and until we can accurately target the patient and timing in which systemic steroids will work effectively with minimal side effects it is essential that parents are involved in decision-making and that these uncertainties are discussed.

## Future directions

Further investigation into the role of inhaled steroids for the ventilator-dependent infant may be valuable, given the potentially different risk benefit profile [108,109]. Intra-tracheal administration of surfactant combined with budesonide in a trial of 265 preterm infants conferred a reduced risk of CLD or death in comparison to controls receiving only surfactant [110].

Alternative methods of ventilation are the subject of ongoing research. Neurally adjusted ventilatory-assist ventilation interprets electrical signals from the diaphragm in the hope of providing better synchrony with the patient's own breathing and a proportional mechanical delivery to patient effort. Little is known about the impact on clinical outcomes, and it is likely that this will be an area for more research in the future [113].

# FAMILY-INTEGRATED CARE

## Family-centred and family-integrated care

Adapting to becoming caregivers in an unfamiliar, uncertain and often unexpected environment can lead to stress and anxiety both long and short term [108–121]. Family-integrated care (FICare) recognises the importance of family in truly holistic care and aims to shift the historical perspective of parents as 'visitors' on the neonatal intensive care unit (NICU) to being primary caregivers and an integral part of the NICU team. **Figure 5.1** demonstrates the principles and interventions through which this can be achieved in clinical practice.

The evidence base for FICare is compelling, much of it long-standing and from low-resource settings. Reduced rates of infection, duration of intravenous therapy and improvements in infant development have been shown as has a significant reduction in length of stay [118,119]. Further research, including randomised controlled trials, assessing the breadth of impact of a formal FICare model have followed and demonstrate reduced stress and anxiety for parents with improved weight gain and breast-feeding at discharge [120–123].

Delivering FICare in its truest form remains challenging. **Figure 5.2** summarises the common barriers. Individual units adopting the FICare model will need to appreciate the barriers within their own unit and aim to address them with staff and parental education, effective communication, resource development, and collaborative problem solving [120].

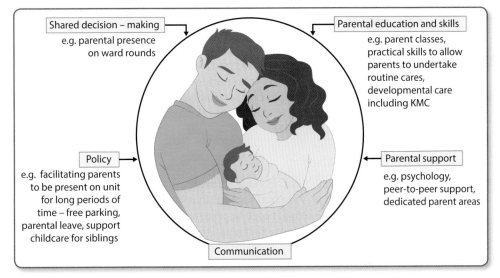

**Figure 5.1** Principles of family-integrated (FI) care and specific interventions.

(KMC, kangaroo mother care)

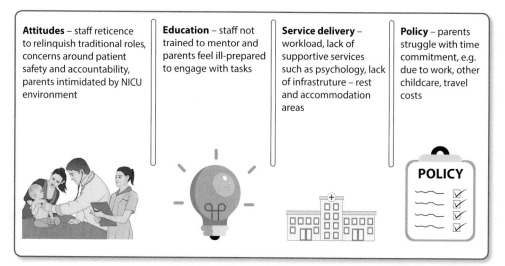

**Attitudes** – staff reticence to relinquish traditional roles, concerns around patient safety and accountability, parents intimidated by NICU environment

**Education** – staff not trained to mentor and parents feel ill-prepared to engage with tasks

**Service delivery** – workload, lack of supportive services such as psychology, lack of infrastructure – rest and accommodation areas

**Policy** – parents struggle with time commitment, e.g. due to work, other childcare, travel costs

POLICY

**Figure 5.2** Barriers to family-integrated (FI) care.
(NICU, neonatal intensive care unit)

## Kangaroo mother care

Kangaroo mother care (KMC) is a specific family-centred intervention classically defined by continuous skin-to-skin contact and feeding exclusively with maternal breast milk [124]. KMC may provide benefit through constant thermal care, tactile stimulation to reduce apnoea, improved breast milk supply, parent–infant bonding and reduced infection risk with less need for invasive procedures and interaction with multiple care providers. KMC originated in Bogotá, Columbia, in 1978 in an attempt to overcome the realities of an overcrowded and under-resourced NICU [125]. Their home KMC programme was reported to reduce morbidity and mortality for low-birth weight infants [125]. General uptake, however, was stymied by concerns around the selection of larger, medically well babies for the intervention [126,127].

Randomised controlled trials (RCTs) strengthening the evidence base have followed and at meta-analysis, KMC is associated with a statistically significant reduction in mortality, length of stay, sepsis rates, along with improved growth indices and exclusive beast-feeding [124,128]. This evidence base largely derives from the low-resource setting, in the context of stable infants with KMC provided by mothers. A recent RCT comparing outcome for 3211 infants randomised to immediate KMC or conventional care until stabilisation, found reduced mortality in the KMC group [129].

## Keeping families together

Common presentations leading to term neonatal admissions include respiratory distress, hypoglycaemia and jaundice [130]. Research suggests that separation of mother and baby soon after birth interrupts essential bonding processes, and can have a detrimental effect on breastfeeding [131–134]. Effective first hour care with early skin-to-skin contact, maintaining normothermia and offering opportunities to feed should be prioritised to reduce term admissions [135]. Transitional care facilities, allowing parents to be resident, and the evolution of community services providing a range of supportive therapies at home have been integral to reducing separation and earlier discharge [136–140].

## Future directions

Research into the impact of interventions that support family-centred care is likely to continue. The impact of KMC in HIC and provision by fathers is interesting; however, there is an argument against over-medicalising an intervention which is clearly family-centred and demonstrates benefit, in favour of pragmatic implementation. Home phototherapy is currently not a commonplace of community service, but it is likely to become more prevalent following evidence supporting its safety profile in select patients and a positive parental experience [141].

# SCREENING

The principles of effective screening remain essentially unchanged since defined by Wilson and Jungner in 1968; identify individuals who appear healthy but are at increased risk of a specific condition, when there is an opportunity to intervene and optimise outcomes. There should be a diagnostic test available, which is acceptable to the group being screened, and infra-structure to support onward treatment [142,143]. There is a great advantage of diagnosis in the neonatal period where early interventions may optimise outcomes for many conditions. In most HIC, mass spectrometry has facilitated cost-effective testing for multiple diseases on a single-dried blood spot sample, though programmes differ between countries [144–148]. With the expansion of programmes there are now examples of diseases which do not fit traditional screening criteria [147].

Screening opportunities are not limited to the newborn bloodspot which is largely only readily available in HIC. Screening mothers for infectious diseases, monitoring infants with risk factors for sepsis and hypoglycaemia all provide an opportunity for early intervention. The routine new-born examination is another opportunity for screening for a multitude of congenital anomalies that can be effectively managed after identification.

Pulse oximetry screening for critical congenital heart disease (CCHD) has a sensitivity of 76.3% and specificity of 99.9% [149]. In the USA, prior to the introduction of universal screening, States that offered this were found to have a higher reduction in CCDH mortality compared to those that did not [151]. On the other hand, in the UK, universal screening has not been mandated by the National Screening Committee due to the risk of false positives, along with a lack of definitive evidence for improved outcomes by diagnosing asymptomatic infants [151,152]. Despite this conclusion a recent survey revealed that 51% of UK units were performing routine screening [153]. There are those exploring routine pulse oximetry screening in LMIC, but this requires access to onward diagnostic and treatment pathways that have the ability to improve outcomes [154–156].

## The future of screening

The research potential of dried blood spot samples has been harnessed by countries such as Denmark which stores left-over specimens, initially taken for screening, in a biobank that can be accessed for research [157,158]. Parents, or patients themselves in due course, can opt out of participation. Estimates suggest up to 37.5% of samples in the biobank have been included in published research [158]. While this provides a rich resource, questions around transparency and the completeness of informed consent have been raised.

The 'Genetic Alliance' (UK) has recommended a trial of whole genome sequencing for newborns at birth [159]. In England, the New-born Genomes Programme will implement a research study to explore offering whole genome sequencing to all newborns as a screening programme to aid rapid diagnosis for rare conditions and ideally improve outcomes [160]. This pilot, projected to include 200,000 babies, will seek to establish whether early diagnosis can be achieved but also aim to evaluate if such a programme will have the benefit of enabling research and new treatments for patients and the possibility of a 'lifetime genomic record' [160]. This raises ethical dilemmas around the implications on wider family members, anxiety that may result from variants of uncertain significance, and how best to manage mutations that reflect genetic susceptibility in the context of multi-factorial conditions or those that lead to disease without effective intervention. Currently, the programme remains in the development stage; at the time of writing they are seeking to establish which genetic conditions and variants should be tested for and shared with parents within the study [160,161]. Without such precision a large yield of variants of unknown significance or pathogenic genes for adult conditions may induce parental worry and resource burden; various groups have recommended that such screening should only be targetting high-risk conditions which can be treated [162,163]. The programme has established four principles with which they will be choosing conditions to target namely, a condition with reliably targetable variants that is debilitating if undiagnosed but can be improved with early intervention where the said intervention is equitably accessible [162]. Many other concerns have been raised by others and are not discussed here; however, the Nuffield Council of Bioethics has provided a briefing note with a discussion of the ethical dilemmas and signposting to relevant academic and policy literature [164]. It is also worth-noting that such a screening test cannot replace the new-born blood-spot screening test for conditions such as congenital hypothyroidism.

## CONCLUSION

Neonatology is a relatively young speciality and there have been many advances in the care of newborn infants, particularly those born preterm, which have been underpinned by research evidence. However there remain many unanswered uncertainties and variation in clinical practice within and between countries. In this chapter, we have focused on care and interventions we believe are relevant globally. However, in high income settings in particular, there have been better nutrition (enteral and parenteral), neuroprotection for both preterm and term infants, pain management and care of infants with surgical conditions and congenital anomalies. Global clinical and research efforts are focused on improving care that will improve not only survival, but also the neurodevelopmental outcomes and quality of life so these infants are able to thrive into child and adulthood.

## REFERENCES

1. World Health Organization. Newborns: improving survival and well-being. © 2020. [cited 2021 October 12th]. Available from https://www.who.int/news-room/fact-sheets/detail/newborns-reducing-mortality. (Last accessed 23rd january 2023).
2. World Health Organization. Born Too Soon: The Global Action Report on Preterm Birth. © 2021. [cited 2021 October 12th]. Available from https://www.who.int/reproductivehealth/publications/maternal_perinatal_health/9789241503433/en/. (Last accessed 23rd january 2023).
3. Steer P. The epidemiology of preterm labour. BJOG 2005; 112:1–3.
4. Denison FC, Aedla NR, Keag O, et al. On behalf of the Royal College of Obstetricians and Gynaecologists. Care of Women with Obesity in Pregnancy: Green-top Guideline No. 72. BJOG. © 2018. [cited 2021 October 12th]. Available from https://www.rcog.org.uk/en/guidelines-research-services/guidelines/gtg72/. (Last accessed 23rd january 2023).

5.  Royal College of Obstetricians and Gynaecologists. The Investigation and Management of the Small-for-Gestational Age Fetus: Green-top Guideline 31. © 2013. [cited 2021 October 12th]. Available from https://www.rcog.org.uk/globalassets/documents/guidelines/gtg_31.pdf. (Last accessed 23rd january 2023).

6.  National Institute of Clinical Excellence (NICE). Antenatal Care. © 2021. [cited 2021 October 12th]. Available from https://www.nice.org.uk/guidance/ng201. (Last accessed 23rd January 2023).

7.  National Institute of Clinical Excellence (NICE). Smoking: stopping in pregnancy and after childbirth. © 2010. [cited 2021 October 12th]. Available from https://www.nice.org.uk/guidance/ph26. (Last accessed 23rd January 2023).

8.  Public Health England. Infectious diseases in pregnancy screening (IDPS): programme overview. © 2015. [cited 2021 October 12th]. Available from https://www.gov.uk/topic/population-screening-programmes/infectious-diseases-in-pregnancy. (Last accessed 23rd January 2023).

9.  National Institute of Clinical Excellence (NICE). Diabetes in pregnancy: management from preconception to the postnatal period. © 2015. [cited 2021 October 12th]. Available from: https://www.nice.org.uk/guidance/ng3. (Last accessed 23rd January 2023).

10. National Institute of Clinical Excellence (NICE). Hypertension in pregnancy: diagnosis and management. © 2019. [cited 2021 October 12th]. Available from https://www.nice.org.uk/guidance/ng133. (Last accessed 23rd January 2023).

11. Roberts D, Brown J, Medley N, Dalziel S. Antenatal corticosteroids for accelerating fetal lung maturation for women at risk of preterm birth. Cochrane Database Syst Rev 2017; 3:CD004454.

12. Doyle L, Crowther C, Middleton P, Marret S, Rouse D. Magnesium sulphate for women at risk of preterm birth for neuroprotection of the fetus. Cochrane Database Syst Rev 2009; CD004661.

13. Althabe F, Belizán J, McClure E, et al. A population-based, multifaceted strategy to implement antenatal corticosteroid treatment versus standard care for the reduction of neonatal mortality due to preterm birth in low-income and middle-income countries: the ACT cluster randomised trial. Lancet 2015; 385:629–639.

14. The WHO ACTION Trials Collaborators. Antenatal Dexamethasone for Early Preterm Birth in Low-Resource Countries. NEJM 2020; 383:2514–2525.

15. WHO. WHO recommendations on antenatal corticosteroids for improving preterm birth outcomes. © 2022. [cited 2023 January 30th]. Available from: https://www.who.int/publications/i/item/9789240057296

16. Chien LY, Whyte R, Aziz K, et al. Improved outcome of preterm infants when delivered in tertiary centres. Obstet Gynecol 2001; 98:247–252.

17. Helenius K, Longford N, Lehtonen L, Modi N, Gale C. Association of early postnatal transfer and birth outside a tertiary hospital with mortality and severe brain injury in extremely preterm infants: observational cohort study with propensity score matching. BMJ 2019; 367.

18. Pan S, Jiang S, Lin S, et al. Reduction of Infection in Neonatal Intensive Care Units using the Evidence-based Practice for Improving Quality (REIN-EPIQ) Study Group. Transl Pediatr 2021; 10:306–314.

19. O'Donnell C, Kamlin C, Davis P, Morley C. Crying and breathing by extremely preterm infants immediately after birth. J Pediatr 2010; 156:846–847.

20. Rabe H, Gyte GM, Díaz-Rossello JL, Duley L. Effect of timing of umbilical cord clamping and other strategies to influence placental transfusion at preterm birth on maternal and infant outcomes. Cochrane Database Syst Rev 2019; CD003248.

21. Madar J, Roehr C, Ainsworth S, et al. European Resuscitation Council Guidelines 2021: Newborn resuscitation and support of transition of infants. Resuscitation 2021; 161:291–326.

22. Ainsworth S, Fawke J. Newborn Life Support, 5th edition. London (UK): Resuscitation Council UK, 2021.

23. Aziz K, Lee H, Escobedo M, et al. Part 5: Neonatal Resuscitation: 2020 American Heart Association Guidelines for Cardiopulmonary Resuscitation and Emergency Cardiovascular Care. Circulation 2020; 142:S524–S550.

24. Wyckoff M, Wyllie J, Aziz K, et al. Neonatal Life Support 2020 International Consensus on Cardiopulmonary Resuscitation and Emergency Cardiovascular Care Science with Treatment Recommendations. Resuscitation 2020; 156:A156–A187.

25. National Institute for Health and Care Excellence (NICE). Specialist neonatal respiratory care for babies born preterm. 2019 NICE guideline. Available from: www.nice.org.uk/guidance/ng124 (Last accessed 23rd january 2023).

26. Sweet DG, Carnielli V, Griersen G, et al. European consensus guidelines on the management of respiratory distress syndrome – 2019 update. Neonatology 2019; 115:432–450.
27. Subramaniam P, Ho J, Davis P. Prophylactic nasal continuous positive airway pressure for preventing morbidity and mortality in very preterm infants. Cochrane Database Syt Rev 2016; 14:CD001243.
28. Waldron S, MacKinnon R. Neonatal thermoregulation. Infant 2002; 3:101–104.
29. Jain A, Fleming P. Project 27/28. Arch Dis Child Fetal Neonatal Ed 2004; 89:F14–F16.
30. Brouwer E, Knol R, Vernooij ASN, et al. Physiological-based cord clamping in preterm infants using a new purpose-built resuscitation table: a feasibility study. Arch Dis Child Fetal Neonatal Ed 2019; 104:F396–F402.
31. Thomas M, Yoxall C, Weeks A, Duley L. Providing newborn resuscitation at the mother's bedside: assessing the safety, usability and acceptability of a mobile trolley. BMC Pediatr 2014; 14:135.
32. Katheria A, Sorkhi S, Hassen K, et al. Acceptability of bedside resuscitation with intact umbilical cord to clinicians and patients families in the United States. Front Pediatr 2018; 6:100.
33. Balasubramanian H, Ananthan A, Jain V, et al. Umbilical cord milking in preterm infants: a systematic review and meta-analysis. Arch Dis Child Fetal Neonatal Ed 2020; 105:572–580.
34. Moore T, Hennessy EM, Myles J, et al. Neurological and developmental outcome in extremely preterm children born in England in 1995 and 2006: the EPICure studies. BMJ 2012; 345:e7961.
35. Bates S, Everett E, Johnston T, et al. Perinatal Management of Extreme Preterm Birth before 27 weeks of gestation: A Framework for Practice. British Association of Perinatal Medicine. © 2019. [cited 2021 October 12th]. Available from https://www.bapm.org/resources/80-perinatal-management-of-extreme-preterm-birth-before-27-weeks-of-gestation-2019. (Last accessed 23rd january 2023).
36. Mehler K, Oberthuer A, Keller T, et al. Survival among infants born at 22 or 23 weeks' gestation following active prenatal and postnatal care. JAMA Pediatrics 2016; 170:671–677.
37. Norman M, Hallberg B, Abrahamsson T, et al. Association between year of birth and 1-year survival among extremely preterm infants in Sweden during 2004-2007 and 2014-2016. JAMA 2019; 321:1188–1199.
38. Patel RM, Rysavy MA, Bell EF, Tyson JE. Survival of Infants Born at Periviable Gestational Ages. Clin Perinatol 2017; 44:287–303.
39. Hack M, Wright LL, Shankaran S, et al. Very-low-birth-weight outcomes of the National Institute of Child Health and Human Development Neonatal Network, November 1989 to October 1990. Am J Obstet Gynecol 1995; 172:457–464.
40. Söderström F, Normann E, Jonsson M, et al. Outcomes of a uniformly active approach to infants born at 22–24 weeks of gestation. Arch Dis Child Fetal Neonatal Ed 2021; 106:413–417.
41. Helenius K, Sjörs G, Shah PS, Modi N, et al on behalf of the International Network for Evaluating Outcomes (iNeo) of Neonates. Survival in Very Preterm Infants: An International Comparison of 10 National Neonatal Networks. Pediatrics 2017; 140.
42. Isayama T. The clinical management and outcomes of extremely preterm infants in Japan: past, present and future. Translational Pediatrics 2019; 8:199–211.
43. Kono Y, Yonemoto N, Nakanishi H, Kusuda S, Fujimura M. Changes in survival and neurodevelopmental outcomes of infants born at <25 weeks' gestation: a retrospective observational study in centres in Japan. BMJ Paediatr Open 2018; 2:e00021.
44. World Health Organization. Preterm Birth. © 2018. [cited 2021 October 12th]. Available from https://www.who.int/news-room/fact-sheets/detail/preterm-birth. (Last accessed 23rd january 2023).
45. Helping Babies Breathe. Healthy Newborn Network. [cited 2021 October 12th]. Available from https://www.healthynewbornnetwork.org/partner/helping-babies-breathe/. (Last accessed 23rd january 2023).
46. Pejovic N, Trevisanuto D, Lubulwa C, et al. Neonatal resuscitation using a laryngeal mask airway: a randomised trial in Uganda. Arch Dis Child 2018; 103:255–260.
47. Pejovic NG, Myrnerts Höök S, Byamugisha J. A randomised trial of laryngeal mask airway in neonatal resuscitation. N Engl J Med 2020; 383:2138–2147.
48. O'Shea JE, Scrivens A, Edwards G, Roehr CC. Safe emergency neonatal airway management: current challenges and potential approaches. Arch Dis Child Fetal Neonatal Ed 2021.
49. Leone T, Rich W, Finer N. Neonatal intubation: success of pediatric trainees. J Pediatr 2005; 146:638–641.

50. Fogalia E, Ades A, Sawyer T, et al. Neonatal Intubation Practice and Outcomes: An International Registry Study. Pediatrics 2019; 143:e2180902.

51. Edwards G, Belkhatir K, Brunton A, et al. Neonatal intubation success rates: four UK units. Arch Dis Child Fetal Neonatal Ed 2020; 105:684.

52. Qureshi M, Kumar M. Laryngeal mask airway versus bag-mask ventilation or endotracheal intubation for neonatal resuscitation. Cochrane Database Syst Rev 2018; 3:CD003314.

53. Kamlin CO, O'Donnell CP, Everest NJ, Davis PG, Morley CJ. Accuracy of clinical assessment of infant heart rate in the delivery room. Resuscitation 2006; 71:319–321.

54. Mizumoto H, Tomataki S, Shibta H, et al. Electrocardiogram shows reliable heart rates much earlier than pulse oximetry during neonatal resuscitation. Pediatr Int 2012; 54:205–207.

55. Preziosi MP, Roig JC, Hargrove N, Burchfield DJ. Metabolic acidemia with hypoxia attenuates the hemodynamic responses to epinephrine during resuscitation in lambs. Crit Care Med 1993; 21:1901–1907.

56. Modest VE, Butterworth JF 4th. Effect of pH and lidocaine on beta-adrenergic receptor binding. Interaction during resuscitation? Chest 1995; 108:1373–1379.

57. Daniel SS, Dawes GS, James LS, Ross BB. Analeptics and the resuscitation of asphyxiated monkeys. Br Med J 1966; 2:562–563.

58. Lokesh L, Kumar P, Narang A. A randomised controlled trial of sodium bicarbonate in neonatal resuscitation – effect on immediate outcome. Resuscitation 2004; 60:219–223.

59. Murki S, Kumar P, Lingappa L, et al. Effect of a single dose of sodium bicarbonate given during neonatal resuscitation at birth and on the acid-base status on the first day of life. J Perinatol 2004; 24:696–699.

60. Sáenz P, Brugada M, de Jongh B, et al. A Survey of Intravenous Sodium Bicarbonate in Neonatal Asphyxia among European Neonatologists: Gaps between Scientific Evidence and Clinical Practice. Neonatology 2011; 99:170–176.

61. Singer RB, Deering RC, Clark JK. The acute effects in man of a rapid intravenous infusion of hypertonic sodium bicarbonate solution. Changes in respiration and output of carbon dioxide. J Clin Inves 1956; 35:245–253.

62. Aschner J, Poland R. Sodium Bicarbonate: Basically Useless Therapy. Pediatrics 2008; 122:831–835.

63. Dainty K, Atkins D, Breckwoldt J, et al. on behalf of the International Liaison Committee on Resuscitation's (ILCOR) Pediatric Neonatal Life Support Task Force. Family presence during resuscitation in paediatric and neonatal cardiac arrest: A systematic review. Resuscitation 2021; 162:20–34.

64. Harvey M, Pattison H. The impact of a father's presence during newborn resuscitation: a qualitative interview study with healthcare professionals. BMJ Open 2013; 3:e002547.

65. Yoxall C, Ayers S, Sawyer A, et al. Providing immediate neonatal care and resuscitation at birth beside the mother: clinicians' views, a qualitative study. BMJ Open 2015; 5:e008494.

66. Zehnder E, Law BHY, Schmölzer GM. Does parental presence affect workload during neonatal resuscitation? Arch Dis Child Fetal Neonatal Ed 2020; 105:559–561.

67. Kuypers K, Lamberska T, Martherus T, et al. The effect of a face mask for respiratory support on breathing in preterm infants at birth. Resuscitation 2019; 144:178–184.

68. Kuypers K, Martherus T, Lamberska T, et al. Reflexes that impact spontaneous breathing of preterm infants at birth: a narrative review. Arch Dis Child Fetal Neonatal Ed 2020; 105:675–679.

69. Dargaville PA, Kamlin COF, Orsini F, et al. Effect of Minimally Invasive Surfactant Therapy vs Sham Treatment on Death or Bronchopulmonary Dysplasia in Preterm Infants with Respiratory Distress Syndrome: The OPTIMIST-A Randomized Clinical Trail. JAMA 2021; 326:2478–2487.

70. Smee N, Boyd D, Conetta H, O'Shea J. Laryngeal mask airway surfactant administration: a case series of 60 infants. Arch Dis Child Fetal Neonatal Ed 2021; 106:342.

71. Lamberska T, Settelmayerova E, Smisek J, et al. Oropharyngeal surfactant can improve initial stabilisation and reduce rescue intubation in infants born below 25 weeks of gestation. Acta Paediatr 2018; 107:73–78.

72. Hillman N, Polglase G, Pillow J, et al. Inflammation and lung maturation from stretch injury in preterm sheep. Am J Physiol Lung Cell Mol Physiol 2011; 300:L232–L241.

73. Bohrer B, Silveira R, Neto E, Procianoy R. Mechanical ventilation of newborns infant changes in plasma pro- and anti-inflammatory cytokines. J Pediatr 2010; 156:16–19.

74.  Javaid A, Morris I. Bronchopulmonary Dysplasia. Paediatrics and Child Health 2017; 28:22–27.
75.  Eber E, Zach MS. Long term sequelae of bronchopulmonary dysplasia (chronic lung disease of infancy). Thorax 2001; 56:317–323.
76.  Hakulinen AL, Heinonen K, Länsimies E, Kiekara O. Pulmonary function and respiratory morbidity in school age children born prematurely and ventilated for neonatal respiratory insufficiency. Pediatr Pulmonol 1990; 8:226–232.
77.  Greenough A, Griffin FJ, Yüksel B. Respiratory morbidity in preschool children born prematurely. Relationship to adverse neonatal events. Acta paediatr 1996; 85:772–777.
78.  Malavoti AM, Bassler D, Arlettaz-Mieth R, et al. Bronchopulmonary dysplasia – impact of severity and timing of diagnosis on neurodevelopment of preterm infants: a retrospective cohort study. BMJ Paediatrics Open 2018; 2:e000165.
79.  Katwyk S, Augustine S, Thébaud B, Thavorn K. Lifetime patient outcomes and healthcare utilization for Bronchopulmonary dysplasia (BPD) and extreme preterm infants: a microsimulation study. BMC paediatrics 2020; 20:136.
80.  Mowitz M, Ayyagari R, Gao W, et al. Health Care Burden of Bronchopulmonary Dysplasia Among Extremely Preterm Infants. Front Pediatr 2019; 7:510.
81.  Downham L, Cerovic S, Lessage C, Leroy S. Mortality in preterm infants with bronchopulmonary dysplasia associated pulmonary hypertension: a systematic literature review. Eur Respir J 2020; 56:3502.
82.  Aldana-Aguiree JC, Pinto M, Featherstone RM. Less invasive surfactant administration versus intubation for surfactant delivery in preterm infants with respiratory distress syndrome: a systematic review and meta-analysis. Arch Dis Child Fetal Neonatal Ed 2017; 102:F17–F23.
83.  Bellos I, Fitrou G, Panza R, Pandita A. Comparative efficacy of methods for surfactant administration: a network meta-analysis. Arch Dis Child Fetal Neonatal Ed 2021.
84.  Vento M, Bohlin K, Herting E, Roehr C, Dargaville P. Surfactant Administration via Thin Catheter: A Practical Guide. Neonatology 2019; 116:211–226.
85.  Dekker J, Lopriore E, van Zanten H, et al. Sedation during minimal invasive surfactant therapy: a randomised controlled trial. Arch Dis Child Fetal Neonatal Ed 2019; 104:F378–F383.
86.  Herting E, Härtel C, Göpel W. Less invasive surfactant administration (LISA): chances and limitations. Arch Dis Child Fetal Neonatal Ed 2019; 104:F655–F659.
87.  Wilkinson D, Andersen C, O'Donnell C, De Paoli A, Manley B. High flow nasal cannula for respiratory support in preterm infants. Cochrane Database Syst Rev 2016; 2:CD006405.
88.  Hong H, Li X, Li J, Zhang Z. High-flow nasal cannula versus nasal continuous positive airway pressure for respiratory support in preterm infants: a meta- analysis of randomized controlled trials. J Matern Fetal Neonatal Med 2021; 34:259–266.
89.  Klingenberg C, Wheeler K, McCalion N, Morley C, Davis P. Volume-targeted versus pressure-limited ventilation in neonates. Cochrane Database Syst Rev 2017; 10:CD003666.
90.  Peng W, Zhu H, Shi H, Liu E. Volume targeted ventilation is more suitable than pressure-limited ventilation for preterm infants: a systematic review and meta-analysis. Arch Dis Child Fetal Neonatal Ed 2014; 99:F158–F165.
91.  Van Wyk L, Tooke L, Dippenaar R, et al. Optimal Ventilation and Surfactant Therapy in Very-Low-Birth-Weight Infants in Resource-Restricted Regions. Neonatology 2020; 117:217–224.
92.  Clark R, Davis S, Visick M, Bell R. Feasibility of bubble continuous positive airway pressure in secondary facilities in low and middle income countries. Med Res Arch 2018; 6:1–8.
93.  Kawaza K, Machen H, Brown J, et al. Efficacy of a low-cost bubble CPAP system in treatment of respiratory distress in a neonatal ward in Malawi. PLoS One 2014; 9:e86327.
94.  Kinshella MLW, Walker C, Hiwa T, et al. Barriers and facilitators to implementing bubble CPAP to improve neonatal health in sub-Saharan Africa: a systematic review. Pub Health Rev 2020; 41:6.
95.  Askie L, Darlow B, Finer N, et al. Association Between Oxygen Saturation Targeting and Death or Disability in Extremely Preterm Infants in the Neonatal Oxygenation Prospective Meta-Analysis Collaboration. JAMA 2018; 319:2190–2201.
96.  Sturrock S, Williams E, Dassios T, Greenough A. Closed loop automated oxygen control in neonates – A review. Acta Paediatr 2020; 109:914–922.

97. Gajdos M, Waitz M, Mendler MR, Braun W, Hummler H. Effects of a new device for automated closed loop control of inspired oxygen concentration on fluctuations of arterial and different regional organ tissue oxygen saturations in preterm infants. Arch Dis Child Fetal Neonatal Ed 2019; 104:F360–F365.

98. Reynolds PR, Miller TL, Volakis LI, et al. Randomised cross-over study of automated oxygen control for preterm infants receiving nasal high flow. Arch Dis Child Fetal Neonatal Ed 2019; 104:F366–F371.

99. Tan K, Lai NM, Jones LJ, Plottier GK, Dargaville P. Automated oxygen delivery for preterm infants with respiratory dysfunction. Cochrane Database Syst Rev 2019; 2019:CD013294.

100. Halliday H. Postnatal steroids: still a dilemma for neonatologists and parents? Arch Dis Child Fetal Neonatal Ed 2018; 103:F500–F502.

101. Ramaswamy VV, Bandyyopadhyay T, Nanda D, et al. Assessment of Postnatal Corticosteroids for the Prevention of Bronchopulmonary Dysplasia in Preterm Neonates. A Systematic Review and Network Meta-analysis. JAMA Pediatr 2021; 175:e206826.

102. Yeh TF, Lin YJ, Huang CC, et al. Early dexamethasone therapy in preterm infants: a follow-up study. Pediatrics 1998; 101:E7.

103. Shinwell ES, Karplus M, Reich D, et al. Early postnatal dexamethasone treatment and increased incidence of cerebral palsy. Arch Dis Child Fetal Neonatal Ed 2000; 83:F177–F181.

104. Doyle L, Davis P, Morley C, McPhee A, Carlin JB. Low-dose dexamethasone facilitates extubation among chronically ventilator-dependent infants: a multicenter, international, randomized, controlled trial. Pediatrics 2006; 117:75–83.

105. Doyle L, Davis P, Morley C, McPhee A, Carlin JB. Outcome at 2 years of age of infants from the DART study: a multicenter, international, randomized, controlled trial of low-dose dexamethasone. Pediatrics 2007; 119:716–721.

106. Doyle L, Cheong J, Ehrenkranz RA, Halliday HL. Late (> 7 days) systemic postnatal corticosteroids for prevention of bronchopulmonary dysplasia in preterm infants. Cochrane Database Syst Rev 2017; 10:CD001145.

107. Onland W, De Jaegere A, Offringa M, van Kaam A. Systemic corticosteroid regimens for prevention of bronchopulmonary dysplasia in preterm infants. Cochrane Database Syst Rev 2017; 1:CD010941.

108. Shah S, Ohlsson A, Halliday H, Shah V. Inhaled versus systemic corticosteroids for the treatment of bronchopulmonary dysplasia in ventilated very low birth weight preterm infants. Cochrane Database Syst Rev 2017; 2017:CD002057.

109. Onland W, Offringa M, van Kaam A. Late (≥ 7 days) inhalation corticosteroids to reduce bronchopulmonary dysplasia in preterm infants. Cochrane Database Syst Rev 2017; 8:CD002311.

110. Yeh T, Chen C, Wu S, et al. Intratracheal Administration of Budesonide/Surfactant to Prevent Bronchopulmonary Dysplasia. Am J Respir Crit Care Med 2016; 193:86–95.

111. Baud O, Maury L, Lebail F, et al. Effect of early low-dose hydrocortisone on survival without bronchopulmonary dysplasia in extremely preterm infants (PREMILOC): a double-blind, placebo-controlled, multicentre, randomised trial. Lancet 2016; 387:1827–1836.

112. Baud O, Trousson C, Biran V, et al. Association Between Early Low-Dose Hydrocortisone Therapy in Extremely Preterm Neonates and Neurodevelopmental Outcomes at 2 Years of Age. JAMA 2017; 317:1329–1337.

113. Rossor T, Hunt K, Shetty S, Greenough A. Neurally adjusted ventilatory assist compared to other forms of triggered ventilation for neonatal respiratory support. Cochrane Database Syst Rev 2017; 10:CD012251.

114. Janvier A, Lantos J, Aschner J, et al. Stronger and more vulnerable: A balanced view of the impacts of the NICU experience on parents. Pediatrics 2016; 138:e20160655.

115. Gallagher K, Shaw C, Aladangady N, Marlow N. Parental experience of interaction with healthcare professionals during their infant's stay in the neonatal intensive care unit. Arch Dis Child Fetal Neonatal Ed 2018; 103:F343–F348.

116. Feeley N, Zelkowitz P, Cormier C, et al. Posttraumatic stress among mothers of very low birthweight infants at 6 months after discharge from the neonatal intensive care unit. Appl Nurs Res 2011; 24:114–117.

117. Shaw RJ, Bernard RS, Storfer-Isser A, et al. Parental coping in the neonatal intensive care unit. J Clin Psychol Med Settings 2013; 20:135–142.

118. Levin A. The Mother-Infant unit at Tallinn Children's Hospital, Estonia: a truly baby-friendly unit. Birth 1994; 21:39–44.
119. Bhutta ZA, Khan I, Salat S, et al. Reducing length of stay in hospital for very low birthweight infants by involving mothers in a stepdown unit: an experience from Karachi (Pakistan). BMJ 2004; 329:1151–1155.
120. Patel N, Ballantyne A, Bowker G, et al. Family Integrated Care: changing the culture in the neonatal unit. Arch Dis Child Fetal Neonatal Ed 2018; 103:415–419.
121. O'Brien K, Robson K, Bracht M, et al. Effectiveness of Family Integrated Care in neonatal intensive care units on infant and parent outcomes: a multicentre, multinational, cluster-randomised controlled trial. Lancet Child Adolesc Health 2018; 2:245–254.
122. O'Brien K, Bracht M, Macdonell K, et al. A pilot cohort analytic study of family integrated care in a Canadian neonatal intensive care unit. BMC Pregnancy Childbirth 2013; 13:S12.
123. Benzies K, Aziz K, Shah V, et al. Effectiveness of Alberta Family Integrated Care on infant length of stay in level II neonatal intensive care units: a cluster randomized controlled trial. BMC Pediatr 2020; 20:535.
124. Conde-Agudelo A, Belizán JM, Diaz-Rossello J. Kangaroo mother care to reduce morbidity and mortality in low birthweight infants. Cochrane Database Syst Rev 2012; 16:CD002771.
125. Charpak N, Ruiz JG, Zupan J, et al. Kangaroo Mother Care: 25 years after. Acta Paediatr 2005; 94:514–522.
126. Whitelaw A, Sleath K. Myth of the marsupial mother: home care of very low birth weight babies in Bogota, Columbia. The Lancet 1985; 1:1206–1208.
127. Simkiss DE. Editorial. Kangaroo mother care. J Trop Paediatr 1999; 45:192–194.
128. Charpak N, Ruiz-Peláez JG, Figueroa de C Z, Charpak Y. Kangaroo mother versus traditional care for newborn infants. Pediatrics 1997; 100:682–688.
129. WHO Immediate KMC Study Group. Immediate Kangaroo Mother Care and Survival of Infants with Low Birth Weight. N Engl J Med 2021; 384:2028–2038.
130. Battersby C, Michaelides S, Upton M, Rennie J. Term admissions to neonatal units in England: a role for transitional care? A retrospective cohort study. BMJ Open 2017; 7:e016050.
131. Leiderman PH, Seashore MJ. Mother-infant neonatal separation: some delayed consequences. Ciba Found Symp 1975; 213–239.
132. Howard K, Martin A, Berlin L, Brooks-Gunn J. Early Mother-Child Separation, Parenting and Child Well-Being in Early Head Start Families. Attach Hum Dev 2011; 13:5–26.
133. Flacking R, Lehtonen L, Thomson G, et al. Closeness and separation in neonatal intensive care. Acta Paediatr 2012; 101:1032–1037.
134. Conti M, Natale F, Stolfi I, et al. Consequences of Early Separation of Maternal-Newborn Dyad in Neonates Born to SARS-CoV-2 Positive Mothers: An Observational Study. Int J Environ Res Public Health 2021; 18:5899.
135. NHS Improvement. Reducing harm leading to avoidable admission of full-term babies into neonatal units. © 2017. [cited 2021 October 17th]. Available from https://www.england.nhs.uk/wp-content/uploads/2021/03/reducing-harm-leading-to-avoidable-admission-of-full-term-babies-into-neonatal-units.pdf. (Last accessed 23rd january 2023).
136. British Association of Perinatal Medicine. Neonatal Transitional Care – A Framework for Practice. © 2017. [cited 2021 October 17th]. Available from https://www.bapm.org/resources/24-neonatal-transitional-care-a-framework-for-practice-2017. (Last accessed 23rd january 2023).
137. Balfour-Lynn IM, Field DJ, Gringras P, et al. BTS guidelines for home oxygen in children. Br Thorac Soc Guidelines Thorax 2009; 64:ii1–26.
138. Lagatta JM, Uhing M, Acharya K, et al. Actual and Potential Impact of a Home Nasogastric Tube Feeding Program for Infants Whose Neonatal Intensive Care Unit Discharge Is Affected by Delayed Oral Feedings. J Pediatr 2021; 234:38–45.
139. Wood K, O'Brien F, Liddle K, Dore R. A neonatal short-term home nasogastric tube feeding programme. Infant 2020; 16.
140. McGill-Vargas L. NICU QI Initiative: Home Nasogastric Tube Feedings. © 2018. [cited 2021 October 17th]. Available from https://wcaap.org/nicu-qi-initiative-home-nasogastric-tube-feedings/ (Last accessed 23rd january 2023).

141. Noureldein M, Mupanemunda G, McDermott H, et al. Home phototherapy for neonatal jaundice in the UK: a single-centre retrospective service evaluation and parental survey. BMJ Paediatrics Open 2021; 5:e001027.

142. NHS. NHS screening. © 2021. [cited 2021 October 17th]. Available from https://www.nhs.uk/conditions/nhs-screening/ (Last accessed 23rd january 2023).

143. Wilson, James Maxwell Glover, Jungner, Gunnar & World Health Organization. Principles and practice of screening for disease. © 1968. [cited 2021 October 17th]. Available from https://apps.who.int/iris/handle/10665/37650. (Last accessed 23rd january 2023).

144. Downing M, Pollitt R. Newborn bloodspot screening in the UK – past, present and future. Ann Clin Biochem 2008; 45:11–17.

145. Guthrie R, Susi A. A Simple Phenylalanine Method For Detecting Phenylketonuria in Large Populations of Newborn Infants. Pediatrics 1963; 32:338–343.

146. Public Health England. PHE Screening. © 2021. [cited 2021 October 17th]. Available from https://phescreening.blog.gov.uk/2020/01/15/blood-spot-screening-50/. (Last accessed 23rd january 2023).

147. Kelly N, Makarem D, Wasserstein M. Screening of Newborns for Disorders with High Benefit-Risk Ratios Should be Mandatory. J Law Med Ethics 2016; 44:231–240.

148. Kerruish N, Robertson S. Newborn screening: new developments, new dilemmas. J Med Ethics 2005; 31:393–398.

149. Plana M, Zamora J, Suresh G, et al. Pulse oximetry screening for critical congenital heart defects. Cochrane Database Syst Rev 2018; 3:CD011912.

150. Abouk R, Grosse SD, Ailes E, et al. Association of US State Implementation of New-born Screening Policies for Critical Congenital Heart Disease with Early Infant Cardiac Deaths. JAMA 2017; 318:2111–2118.

151. Ewer A, Deshpande S, Gale C, et al. Potential benefits and harms of universal pulse oximetry screening: response to the UK National Screening Committee public consultation. Arch Dis Child 2020; 105:1128–1129.

152. UK National Screening Committee. Consultation on the use of pulse oximetry as an additional test in the Newborn and Infant Physical Exam. © 2019. [cited 2021 October 17th]. Available from https://legacyscreening.phe.org.uk/documents/pulse-oximetry/Consultation%20covernote%202019.pdf. (Last accessed 23rd january 2023).

153. Brown S, Liyanage S, Mikrou P, Singh A, Ewer AK. Newborn pulse oximetry screening in the UK: a 2020 survey. The Lancet 2020; 396:881.

154. Zheleva B, Nair S, Dobrzycka A, Saarinen A. Considerations for Newborn Screening for Critical Congential Heart Disease in Low- and Middle-Income Countries. Int J Neonatal Screen 2020; 6:49.

155. Hom L, Martin G. Newborn Critical Congenital Heart Disease Screening Using Pulse Oximetry: Value and Unique Challenges in Developing Regions. Int J Neonatal Screen 2020; 6:74.

156. Van Niekerk AM, Cullis RM, Linley LL, Zühlke L. Feasibility of Pulse Oximetry Pre-Discharge Screening Implementation for Detecting Critical Congenital Heart Lesions in Newborns in a Secondary Level Maternity Hospital in the Western Cape, South Africa: The 'POPSICLe' Study. S Afr Med J 2016; 106:817.

157. Statens Serum Institute. The Danish Neonatal Screening Biobank (DNSB). [cited 2021 October 17th]. Available from https://www.ssi.dk/-/media/arkiv/dk/sygdomme-beredskab-og-forskning/screening-af-medfoedte-sygdomme/the-danish-neonatal-screening-biobank-07082015.pdf?la=da. (Last accessed 23rd january 2023).

158. Hougaard D, Bybjerg-Grauholm J, Christiansen M, Nørgaard-Pedersen. Response to 'Newborn dried blood spot samples in Denmark: the hidden figures of secondary use and research participation. Eur J Hum Genet 2019; 27:1625–1627.

159. NHS Health Education England. Newborn screening: time to expand the list? © 2019. [cited 2021 October 17th]. Available from https://www.genomicseducation.hee.nhs.uk/blog/newborn-screening-time-to-expand-the-list/ (Last accessed 23rd january 2023).

160. Genomics England. Newborn Genomes Programme. July 2021. Available from https://www.genomicsengland.co.uk/initiatives/newborns (Last accessed 23rd january 2023).

161. Genomics England. Choosing conditions. Available from https://www.genomicsengland.co.uk/initiatives/newborns/choosing-conditions (Last accessed 23 january 2023).

162. Friedman JM, Cornel MC, Goldenberg AJ, et al. Genomic newborn screening: public health policy considerations and recommendations. BMC Med Genomics 2017; 10:9.

163. Howard H, Knoppers B, Cornel M, et al. Whole-genome sequencing in newborn screening? A statement on the continued importance of targeted approached in newborn screening programmes. Eur J Hum Genet 2015; 23:1593–1600.

164. Nuffield Council on Bioethics. Whole genome sequencing of babies. 2018. Available from https://www.nuffieldbioethics.org/publications/whole-genome-sequencing-of-babies/briefing-note/ethical-issues (Last accessed 23rd january 2023).

# Chapter 6

# Management of musculo-skeletal problems in cerebral palsy based on motor function – using the gross motor function classification system

*Ken Ye, Erich Rutz, Abhay Khot*

## BACKGROUND

Cerebral palsy (CP) is the most common cause of disability in children, affecting approximately 1 in 500 newborns across the globe [1]. CP describes a group of permanent disorders of movement and posture that are attributed to non-progressive disturbances in the developing fetal or infant brain that affects motor, sensory, cognition and behaviour [2]. While the initial brain injury is non-progressive, the clinical manifestations affecting the musculoskeletal (MSK) system are progressive and relate to significant pathology in body structure and disability affecting function. The management of these problems must be tailored to the needs of the child at each stage of development to maximise and maintain the functional capacity of each child. The Gross Motor Function Classification System (GMFCS) and the most recent classification for musculoskeletal pathology (MSP) help to classify and guide our management based on natural history and functional profiles of children with CP [3,4].

The GMFCS stratifies CP into five levels of function from GMFCS I to GMFCS V [2]. This system helps to guide management strategies, and set goals of treatment for each level,

**Ken Ye** MBBS BMedSci PhD FRACS (Ortho), Paediatric Orthopaedic Department, The Royal Children's Hospital, Parkville, Australia
Email: mr.yekken@gmail.com

**Erich Rutz** MD PhD PD FRACS (Ortho), Paediatric Orthopaedic Department, The Royal Children's Hospital, Parkville; Department of Paediatrics, Bob Dickens Chair for Paediatric Orthopaedic Surgery, The University of Melbourne; Hugh Williamson Gait Analysis Laboratory, The Royal Children's Hospital; Murdoch Children's Research Institute, Melbourne, Australia; Medical Faculty, University of Basel, Basel, Switzerland
Email: erich_rutz@hotmail.com

**Abhay Khot** MS DNB FRCS (Tr & Orth) FRACS, Paediatric Orthopaedic Department, The Royal Children's Hospital, Parkville, Australia
Email: abhay.khot@rch.org.au

and importantly, highlights the natural progression of function of each level. This natural history is important in guiding the clinician in therapy and the family in understanding expectations. Therefore, the GMFCS is a grading system and not an outcome measure. However, the GMFCS level of the child correlates well with the prevalence and severity of medical and orthopaedic conditions and allows us to predict potential issues that may arise in the treatment of such children [5,6].

The progressive nature of the orthopaedic manifestation of CP makes management challenging for the orthopaedic surgeon, both in choosing what intervention to recommend as well as the timing of such interventions. Rang et al (1990) proposed a scheme to describe the musculoskeletal staging into three stages of spasticity, followed by contractures then finally bony deformities [2]. Based on these concepts, Graham et al (2021) recently published the MSP classification system which combines the four stages of hypertonia, contractures, bony deformity, and decompensation, with pathology experience at each anatomical level and the subsequent management options for each stage [3].

The overall management of children with CP is complex and requires a multi-disciplinary team for optimal outcomes. The goals of treatment should be to improve and maintain function and quality of life for these children and allowing them to maximise their full potential. At the very least, we must ensure our interventions, respect the natural development of their condition and we must not 'harm' the child by offering the wrong intervention at the wrong time. Subsequent sections will focus on the musculoskeletal management based on each GMFCS level. A summary of the impairments and interventions for each GMFCS level is presented in **Table 6.1**.

**Table 6.1. Summary of typical impairments and interventions for each gross motor function classification system (GMFCS) level**

**GMFCS I**

| | Impairments | Interventions |
|---|---|---|
| Spine | Low risk for scoliosis | Usually not required |
| Limb/Gait | LLD | • Orthotics<br>• Epiphysiodesis |
| Hip displacement | Low risk | Surveillance |
| Knee | Low risk for deformities | Usually not required |
| Foot and ankle | Calf contractures | • BoNT-A, physiotherapy when younger<br>• Calf lengthening surgery when older<br>• Orthotics, AFO |

**GMFCS II**

| | Impairments | Interventions |
|---|---|---|
| Spine | Low risk for scoliosis | Usually not required |
| Limb/Gait | LLD<br>Torsional deformities | Multi-level surgery<br>• Re-alignment surgery<br>• De-rotation osteotomies of femur, tibia<br>• Guided growth |

*Continues opposite*

| Table 6.1. *Continued* | | |
|---|---|---|
| Hip displacement | Low risk | Surveillance |
| Knee | Low risk for deformities | Usually not required |
| Foot and ankle | • Calf contractures<br>• Foot deformities | Foot correction surgery |
| **GMFCS III** | | |
|  | **Impairments** | **Interventions** |
| Spine | Low risk for scoliosis | Usually not required |
| Limb/Gait | • Torsional deformities<br>• Crouch gait | • Avoidance of crouch gait<br>• Multi-level surgery |
| Hip displacement | Moderate risk | • Surveillance<br>• Hip surgery for containment<br>  – Femoral varus and derotation osteotomy<br>  – Pelvic osteotomy |
| Knee | • Flexion deformity<br>• Hamstring contracture and spasticity | • Correction of knee flexion<br>• Distal femoral extension osteotomy<br>• Guided growth |
| Foot and ankle | • Calf contractures<br>• Weakness<br>• Foot deformities | • Foot correction surgery<br>• Stabilisation of distal lever arm<br>• Correction of distal alignment |
| **GMFCS IV and V** | | |
|  | **Impairments** | **Interventions** |
| Spine | Scoliosis | Posterior spinal fusion |
| Limb/Gait | Deformities | • Minimal ambulation requirements<br>• Not for gait correction surgery |
| Hip displacement | High risk | Hip surgery for containment<br>• Adductor release<br>• Open reduction<br>• Femoral and pelvic osteotomies |
| Knee | • Flexion deformities<br>• Hamstring contracture and spasticity | Hamstring release or transfer to improve sitting |
| Foot and ankle | Foot deformities | Foot correction surgery to enable bracing and positioning |

Impairments and interventions also change over time according to the child's development, and this must be taken into account when deciding the most appropriate intervention

(AFO, ankle foot orthosis; BoNT-A, botulinum toxin; LLD, leg length discrepancy)

# GROSS MOTOR FUNCTION CLASSIFICATION SYSTEM I

The GMFCS I children can walk and run without any assistance and climb stairs without the use of railings. Speed, balance, or coordination may be limited but these children function at a very high level. Except for the risk of epilepsy, these children have few medical comorbidities, good levels of intellectual function and have a normal life expectancy. There is almost no risk of spastic hip displacement. Tone management at early stages can be managed with botulinum toxin (BoNT-A) injections and physical therapy.

The most common orthopaedic management for GMFCS I children is for equinus contractures of the gastrocsoleus complex. At an early stage, this can be the managed by using BoNT-A injections, physiotherapy and the use of an ankle-foot orthosis (AFO). Contractures can be assessed using the Silfverskiold test to determine the amount of contracture from the gastrocnemius and soleus respectively and this translates where the calf lengthening surgery can be made [7]. In general, calf-lengthening surgery is divided into zones, from proximal to distal.

Zone 1 involves lengthening the gastrocnemius muscle and includes the Baumann or the Strayer procedure. The Baumann procedure is largely historical in its use as it offers minimal lengthening of the gastrocsoleus complex [7]. The Strayer is a distal gastrocnemius recession that selectively lengthens the gastrocnemius. The Strayer can be combined with a soleal-fascial lengthening (SFL) which provides a 2:1 ratio lengthening of the gastrocnemius and soleus.

Zone 2 lengthening involves gastrocsoleus recession for moderate degree of fixed contracture. This can be performed through a Vulpius or Baker procedure, which releases the conjoined gastrocnemius aponeurosis and soleus fascia. Lengthening here is not selective for either the gastrocnemius or soleus.

Zone 3 lengthening of the Achilles tendon (TAL) is the most powerful. This can be performed using several techniques such as the White slide or a Z-lengthening. While this is very powerful in its correction of an equinus contracture, it also has the highest risk of inducing excessive length in the gastrocsoleus complex and subsequent weakness in ankle plantar flexion. This is therefore in most cases contraindicated in diplegia CP where over-lengthening the calf can result in the development of crouch gait.

## GROSS MOTOR FUNCTION CLASSIFICATION SYSTEM II

The GMFCS II children can walk independently or with some physical assistance, handheld mobility device or use wheeled mobility for longer distances. There is a mild risk of spastic hip displacement (15%). Compared to GMFCS I hemiplegia, GMFCS II tends to have more proximal involvement including knee and hip contractures. Typically, there may be fixed flexion of the knee, fixed flexion, internal rotation and adduction contractures of the hip, in addition to equinovarus or valgus of the foot and ankle. Rotational deformities of the lower limb are also more common with internal femoral torsion and external tibial torsion (ETT) more prevalent in this category.

Gait analysis becomes more important in the diagnosis and management of children in this category because deformities and gait disturbances occur at multiple levels, and it is imperative to diagnose and differentiate between primary effects of the brain lesion, such as hypertonia, etc. secondary changes in the MSK system, and tertiary compensatory mechanisms. With the correct prescription and dose, multiple level surgery (MLS) in this group can help to correct hip displacement, improve alignment, and correct gait dysfunction to improve the efficiency of gait and prevent further deterioration of MSP [8]. This optimises the biomechanical alignment of the lower limbs and protects joint health to enable children to function independently throughout their later childhood and into their young adult lives. Subsequent discussion will include an outline of surgical management options of the lower limb at each level, starting with the foot and ankle.

## Foot and ankle

Spastic equinovarus deformities are common and can cause pain, tripping, brace intolerance and callosities [9]. Clinical examination should also assess for the contribution of muscle and tendon imbalance that is contributing to the deformity and therefore tailor treatment accordingly. This examination may need to be performed under anaesthesia at the time of surgery to further fine-tune the surgical dose. In principle, overactive muscles can be lengthened or transferred, and therefore soft-tissue surgery to correct the varus deformity can include intra-muscular tenotomy of the tibialis posterior, transfer of the tibialis posterior, transfer of the tibialis anterior or a combination of these procedures. In general, children with diplegia are at risk of over-correction to valgus and children with hemiplegia the risk is recurrent equinovarus. Bony surgery may be required for fixed deformities. This includes a lateral closing wedge calcaneal osteotomy or heel shift for hindfoot varus. Calcaneocuboid shortening or fusion is useful to correct adductus and supination.

Equinus can lead to excessive forefoot loading and breaching of the midfoot, resulting in pes equino-plano-valgus deformity. Again, symptoms include pain, callosities especially over the head of the talus, inability to tolerate bracing, culminating in an inefficient lever arm for gait. Clinically, the corrigibility of the deformity is crucial with particular attention to the restoration of the medial arch and reduction of the navicular on the talus. Surgery should aim to stabilise the midfoot and correct deformity through a lateral column lengthening procedure such as os calcis lengthening or extra-articular fusion of the subtalar joint [10–12]. Os calcis lengthening preserves subtalar motion but requires a flexible joint prior to surgery and is generally preferred in independent walkers at GMFCS I and II. At GMFCS III and IV levels, with more severe involvement, a sub-talar fusion is more useful in correcting deformity.

## Tibia

External tibial torsion causes an inefficient level arm of the foot which becomes shortened and maldirected. De-rotation osteotomy through a supra-malleolar osteotomy (SMO) can be used to correct this deformity. An osteotomy 1–2 cm proximal to the distal tibia physis and subsequently fixed using a plate, increases the bony contact area allowing for greater union, stability, and earlier weight-bearing. This may be combined with a fibula osteotomy if larger correction is required. It is important to recognise other factors that contribute to overall foot progression angle, including deformities of the foot and ankle such as pes valgus deformities and proximal deformities of the femur. Correction of the ETT, therefore, forms only part of overall limb alignment surgery.

## Knee

The primary gait disturbances around the knee include stiffness and excessive flexion. Soft-tissue factors that contribute can include spasticity or contractures of the quadriceps or hamstrings. Occasionally, joint contractures also contribute to a fixed flexion deformity of the knee. Surgical options aim to improve knee range and reduced flexion deformities. The management of a flexed knee gait as described by Young et al (2010) includes BoNT-A for hamstring spasticity, distal hamstring lengthening for contractures, rectus or semi-tendinosis transfers and supra-condylar extension osteotomies (SEO), which may also be performed in conjunction with patellar tendon shortening [13]. Guided growth of the distal femur, if remaining growth allows, using either anterior plates or screws can also improve knee extension over time.

## Hip

Hip-flexion contractures can be treated with lengthening of the psoas tendon. For ambulatory patients this is usually done proximally at the brim of the pelvis as this causes less weakness than if released from the lesser trochanter [14]. Most hip procedures involve treatment of either hip displacement and/or rotational malalignment. Proximal femoral osteotomies can be used to de-rotate the femur, adjust NSA through variation, and alter flexion and extension of the distal segment. Pelvic osteotomies may also be required to re-construct the acetabulum. This will be further discussed in further sections.

# GROSS MOTOR FUNCTION CLASSIFICATION SYSTEM III

The GMFCS III children can ambulate in the community with assistance. In addition to spasticity and movement disorders such as dystonia, weakness becomes a major feature in the limitations of function for these children [15,16]. Similar musculoskeletal pathologies exist at GMFCS III level as in GMFCS II, but they may be more severe. Hip pathology becomes more common as almost half of children will have spastic hip displacement that requires surgical intervention. Routine hip surveillance is important in all children with CP, but most relevant for higher GMFCS levels. Younger children with hip displacement or adduction contractures can be treated with preventative procedures such as adductor releases [17].

Crouch gait can be a significant problem for GMFCS III level children. The majority are due to previously over lengthened gastrocsoleus complex [18,19]. However, some are due to the natural history of spastic diplegia. It is important to try to distinguish between the causes of crouch gait, as some causes can be treated surgically, and some cannot. Chronic overload of the extensor mechanism can lead to patella alta and stress fractures of the patella.

The principles of treating crouch gait involve shortening of long knee extensors, correction of knee flexion deformity and correction of all lever arm deformities. The combination of distal femoral extension osteotomy (DFEO) with patella tendon shortening is a powerful method to correct severe crouch gait [20]. In younger children with crouch gait, hamstring surgery and distal femur growth modulation can be used for a more gradual correction of knee extension ability.

# GROSS MOTOR FUNCTION CLASSIFICATION SYSTEM IV

The GMFCS IV children use wheeled mobility in most settings, with some able to walk short distances at home with assistance or a body support walker. The prevalence and severity of medical conditions are increased as well as issues with tone and movement disorders. Management of hip disorders predominates with 70% of these children having moderate to severe hip displacement that requires surgery. The goals of intervention are to allow comfortable sitting, sleeping, personal care and maintain ability to stand for transfers.

Reconstructive hip surgery should be the gold standard of care. Early hip migration should be monitored closely and intervention implemented prior to complete hip dislocation or destruction. Migration percentage of >40% is an indication for surgery [21]. The minimum age for surgery is approximately 4 years, although ideally surgery should be performed when the child is older after the age of 8 years due to size, weight and factors related to medical fitness for surgery. Any reconstructive hip surgery requires optimisation pre-operatively, considering these children often have severe respiratory, neurological, and gastrointestinal conditions.

There are three main components to surgery: (1) adductor release, (2) femoral osteotomy and (3) pelvic osteotomy. The surgical goals are to reduce the displacement and maintain congruent alignment with good stability and symmetric range of motion. This is to achieve pain-free range of motion, adequate range positioning, and encourage stable hip development. Abduction range should be maximised with a medial hip release of the adductors. Femoral correction often requires varus de-rotation and shortening of the proximal femur to correct the NSA to approximately 100° and anterversion to about 10° [22]. The osteotomy often includes resection of the lesser trochanter along with the psoas attachment. Pelvic osteotomies can be used to correct acetabular dysplasia with the San Diego, Dega type osteotomies more commonly used for CP [23,24]. Computed tomography (CT) scans are often used to assess morphology of the femur and acetabulum to guide surgical intervention and direction of pelvic osteotomy. In older children, triple or peri-acetabular osteotomies may be required instead [25].

# GROSS MOTOR FUNCTION CLASSIFICATION SYSTEM V

The GMFCS V children use wheelchair mobility and have limited ability to maintain anti-gravity head and trunk posture. To achieve a comfortable sitting position, they require a straight spine, level pelvis, flexible hips with >90° of flexion and within 30° of full extension. Feet need to be able to rest in the foot plate of the wheelchair. Most of orthopaedic interventions are therefore aimed at scoliosis correction and hip and pelvis surgery to achieve those goals.

In addition to the hip surgery already discussion, scoliosis surgery is required for a straight spine and sometimes also required for pelvic obliquity. Scoliosis in GMFCS IV and V patients presents earlier and progresses more rapidly. GMFCS level is the single strongest predictor of spinal deformity in children with CP [26]. Most non-operative measures are not effective and bracing is also poorly tolerated and does not avoid progression of curve [27]. Major scoliosis surgery needs to be assessed pre-operatively with a multi-disciplinary team for medical and anaesthetic optimisation, including optimisation of nutritional status, gastroesophageal reflux, and lung function. Posterior fusion using either traditional instrumentation or bipolar fixation is the mainstay treatment for scoliosis correction. Fusion to the pelvis is recommended, especially if pelvic obliquity exceeds 10–15° [27,28]. Without fusion the pelvic obliquity may continue to progress. It can be difficult, however, to determine how much of pelvic obliquity is supra-pelvic and how much is pelvic or infra-pelvic.

Outcomes of spinal surgery are effective in correcting curvature, improve sitting position and upper limb function, eating and respiratory function. There are also reported benefits to prolonging life [29].

## CONCLUSION

The orthopaedic management of CP can be challenging and must be tailored at each stage of the child's development to optimise their function. The GMFCS helps to guide our approach towards this goal and has become a system widely used in CP surgery as a framework for discussion around interventions that may improve the lives of children with CP.

## REFERENCES

1. Graham HK, Rosenbaum P, Paneth N, et al. Cerebral palsy. Nat Rev Dis Primers 2016; 2:15082.
2. Rosenbaum P, Paneth N, Leviton A, et al. A report: the definition and classification of cerebral palsy April 2006. Dev Med Child Neurol Suppl 2007; 109:8–14.
3. Graham HK, Thomason P, Willoughby K, et al. Musculoskeletal Pathology in Cerebral Palsy: A Classification System and Reliability Study. Children (Basel) 2021; 8:252.
4. Rosenbaum PL, Walter SD, Hanna SE, et al. Prognosis for gross motor function in cerebral palsy: creation of motor development curves. JAMA 2002; 288:1357–1363.
5. Shevell MI, Dagenais L, Hall N, Consortium R. Comorbidities in cerebral palsy and their relationship to neurologic subtype and GMFCS level. Neurology 2009; 72:2090–2096.
6. Robin J, Graham HK, Selber P, et al. Proximal femoral geometry in cerebral palsy: a population-based cross-sectional study. J Bone Joint Surg Br 2008; 90:1372–1379.
7. Rutz E, McCarthy J, Shore BJ, et al. Indications for gastrocsoleus lengthening in ambulatory children with cerebral palsy: a Delphi consensus study. J Child Orthop 2020; 14:405–414.
8. Graham HK, Baker R, Dobson F, Morris ME. Multilevel orthopaedic surgery in group IV spastic hemiplegia. J Bone Joint Surg Br 2005; 87:548–555.
9. Michlitsch MG, Rethlefsen SA, Kay RM. The contributions of anterior and posterior tibialis dysfunction to varus foot deformity in patients with cerebral palsy. J Bone Joint Surg Am 2006; 88:1764–1768.
10. Mosca VS. Calcaneal lengthening for valgus deformity of the hindfoot. Results in children who had severe, symptomatic flatfoot and skewfoot. J Bone Joint Surg Am 1995; 77:500–512.
11. Dogan A, Zorer G, Mumcuoglu EI, Akman EY. A comparison of two different techniques in the surgical treatment of flexible pes planovalgus: calcaneal lengthening and extra-articular subtalar arthrodesis. J Pediatr Orthop B 2009; 18:167–175.
12. Davids JR. The foot and ankle in cerebral palsy. Orthop Clin North Am 2010; 41:579–593.
13. Young JL, Rodda J, Selber P, Rutz E, Graham HK. Management of the knee in spastic diplegia: what is the dose? Orthop Clin North Am 2010; 41:561–577.
14. Novacheck TF, Trost JP, Schwartz MH. Intramuscular psoas lengthening improves dynamic hip function in children with cerebral palsy. J Pediatr Orthop 2002; 22:158–164.
15. Graham HK. Botulinum toxin type A management of spasticity in the context of orthopaedic surgery for children with spastic cerebral palsy. Eur J Neurol 2001; 8:30–39.
16. Rodda JM, Graham HK, Carson L, Galea MP, Wolfe R. Sagittal gait patterns in spastic diplegia. J Bone Joint Surg Br 2004; 86:251–258.
17. Silver RL, Rang M, Chan J, de la Garza J. Adductor release in nonambulant children with cerebral palsy. J Pediatr Orthop 1985; 5:672–677.
18. Rodda JM, Graham HK, Nattrass GR, et al. Correction of severe crouch gait in patients with spastic diplegia with use of multilevel orthopaedic surgery. J Bone Joint Surg Am 2006; 88:2653–2664.
19. McGinley JL, Dobson F, Ganeshalingam R, et al. Single-event multilevel surgery for children with cerebral palsy: a systematic review. Dev Med Child Neurol 2012; 54:117–128.
20. Stout JL, Gage JR, Schwartz MH, Novacheck TF. Distal femoral extension osteotomy and patellar tendon advancement to treat persistent crouch gait in cerebral palsy. J Bone Joint Surg Am 2008; 90:2470–2484.

21. Rutz E, Vavken P, Camathias C, et al. Long-term results and outcome predictors in one-stage hip reconstruction in children with cerebral palsy. J Bone Joint Surg Am 2015; 97:500–506.

22. Beauchesne R, Miller F, Moseley C. Proximal femoral osteotomy using the AO fixed-angle blade plate. J Pediatr Orthop 1992; 12:735–740.

23. McNerney NP, Mubarak SJ, Wenger DR. One-stage correction of the dysplastic hip in cerebral palsy with the San Diego acetabuloplasty: results and complications in 104 hips. J Pediatr Orthop 2000; 20:93–103.

24. Miller F, Girardi H, Lipton G, et al. Reconstruction of the dysplastic spastic hip with peri-ilial pelvic and femoral osteotomy followed by immediate mobilization. J Pediatr Orthop 1997; 17:592–602.

25. Clohisy JC, Barrett SE, Gordon JE, Delgado ED, Schoenecker PL. Periacetabular osteotomy in the treatment of severe acetabular dysplasia. Surgical technique. J Bone Joint Surg Am 2006; 88:65–83.

26. Soo B, Howard JJ, Boyd RN, et al. Hip displacement in cerebral palsy. J Bone Joint Surg Am 2006; 88:121–129.

27. Miller F. Spinal deformity secondary to impaired neurologic control. J Bone Joint Surg Am 2007; 143–147.

28. Tsirikos AI, Lipton G, Chang WN, Dabney KW, Miller F. Surgical correction of scoliosis in pediatric patients with cerebral palsy using the unit rod instrumentation. Spine (Phila Pa 1976) 2008; 33:1133–1140.

29. Mercado E, Alman B, Wright JG. Does spinal fusion influence quality of life in neuromuscular scoliosis? Spine (Phila Pa 1976) 2007; 32:S120–S125.

# Chapter 7

# Osteoporosis in children – what the paediatrician needs to know?

*Sophia Sakka*

## INTRODUCTION

Bone health of children can be affected by various factors including lifestyle, nutrition, physical activity, genetics, illnesses and medication. Low bone mass attainment during childhood is a risk factor for subsequent fractures and increases the risk of osteoporosis in late adult life. Therefore, maximal bone mass attainment during early life is of critical significance. Osteoporosis is an important but often underappreciated issue in childhood. Paediatricians and general practitioners are the first ones to encounter children at risk of developing secondary osteoporosis or with features of primary osteoporosis. Early recognition and referral to specialists for management of paediatric osteoporosis will give children the chance to treat vertebral or long-bone fractures, prevent future fractures and alter conditions that influence bone mass. They are also advocates of healthy lifestyle to build stronger bones.

This chapter will define osteoporosis in children and will highlight conditions with increased risk for the development osteoporosis. The aim is to provide general paediatricians, as well as specialists, with knowledge regarding conditions that could negatively affect children's bone health and to identify early signs of osteoporosis in children who are at risk and have limited potential of self-recovering fractures. This should result in better monitoring of these children, prevention and management of osteoporosis. It will also give clues to distinguish between non-accidental injury and low-impact fractures caused by primary osteoporosis conditions.

## DEFINITION OF OSTEOPOROSIS

Criteria for the diagnosis of paediatric osteoporosis include the presence of low trauma vertebral fractures alone or the combination of low bone mineral density and several long-bone fractures. In 2013, the International Society of Clinical Densitometry Task Force produced 'Paediatric Positions' that define paediatric osteoporosis [1]. Based on these

**Sophia Sakka** MD PhD, Consultant in Paediatric Endocrinology, Diabetes and Bone, Division of Endocrinology, Metabolism and Diabetes, First Department of Pediatrics, National and Kapodistrian University of Athens, Medical School, 'Aghia Sophia' Children's Hospital, Athens, Greece, Honorary Senior Lecturer, King's College London, UK
Email: sophiasakka.endo@gmail.com

positions, osteoporosis in children is defined by the presence of a clinically significant fracture (i.e. vertebral fracture, VF) or a significant fracture history and a low-bone mineral density (BMD). Vertebral fractures can be scored using the Genant semi-quantitative technique [2]. These positions emphasise the importance of recognising vertebral fractures that can be asymptomatic or can present even with a normal bone density. These are the official position statements for the definition of osteoporosis:

- The finding of one or more vertebral compression fractures is indicative of osteoporosis in the absence of local disease or high energy trauma regardless of the BMD Z-score.
- In the absence of vertebral fractures, the diagnosis of osteoporosis is indicated by both the presence of a clinically significant fracture and BMD Z-score ≤ –2. Clinically, significant fractures are either:
  - Two or more long-bone fractures by age 10 years
  - Three or more long-bone fractures at any age up to 19 years

A more contemporary view of the definition of osteoporosis balances the role of BMD in the paediatric fracture assessment with other important clinical features, including fracture characteristics, the clinical context and, where appropriate, the underlying genetic aetiology [3].

## DIAGNOSIS OF OSTEOPOROSIS

Based on the above definition, a thorough history taking regarding the mechanism of trauma is necessary. A low-trauma fracture is defined as the one caused by fall from a standing height and with low impact forces. Vertebral fractures can be assessed either on plain X-rays or via 'vertebral fracture assessment, VFA' by dual-energy X-ray absorptiometer (DXA). VFA is a very low-radiation approach, especially useful in children who will require monitoring with multiple spine assessments (**Figure 7.1**). Bone mineral

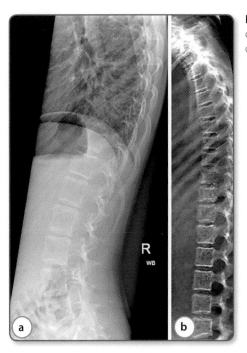

**Figure 7.1** Plain X-ray (a) and VFA (b) of the spine of a patient. VFA can provide a much clearer view of the spine. (from personal files of Dr Sakka).

density in children is calculated in the lumbar spine (LS) or whole body less head (WBLH). Nevertheless, in 2019, the utility of DXA assessment at the forearm, proximal femur, and lateral distal femur was highlighted, especially in children where DXA of LS or whole body is not feasible [4]. In children with short stature and, therefore, smaller bone size, height adjustments need to be performed, in order not to underestimate BMD [5,6]. Based on the latest definition, the focus in paediatric osteoporosis has shifted from bone mineral density alone, to the presence of fractures, especially vertebral fractures.

## Primary osteoporosis

Primary osteoporosis in children covers a range of bone fragility conditions that have a genetic origin. Osteogenesis imperfecta (OI) is an inherited disorder of connective tissue resulting from abnormal quantity and/or quality of type I collagen, the major protein of bone. It accounts for the majority of primary osteoporosis cases. The diagnosis of OI is made based on a clinical history of multiple low impact fractures, along with hypermobility, blue sclerae, skeletal deformities, dentinogenesis imperfecta on clinical examination, and is supported by a positive family history and other investigations, such as imaging techniques, genetic analysis and histology [7]. The traditional Sillence classification of four types of OI, based on severity [8], has now been extended, as new genes responsible for OI keep emerging, some of which have unique characteristics [9]. Therefore, genetic analysis with specific panels for OI can be diagnostic, even though there is still a number of cases with unrecognised mutations.

Rarer forms of primary osteoporosis can also occur and should be suspected in a child with low bone density, long bone and vertebral fractures and no other causative factors, when OI has been excluded. In that case, concordant features, specific for each condition should be sought, such as vision loss in Osteoporosis–Pseudoglioma syndrome.

Idiopathic juvenile osteoporosis is a diagnosis of exclusion. It classically presents with vertebral and metaphyseal fractures in the prepubertal period, back pain and sometimes difficulties walking. In most cases patients experience complete recovery within 3–4 years, after the completion of puberty, but some might remain with residual deformities [10].

## How to differentiate non-accidental injury from osteogenesis imperfecta?

When a child presents with unexplained or low impact fractures, non-accidental injury (NAI) needs to be suspected. Nevertheless, OI should be part of the differential diagnosis. Below are some questions to be asked [11,12]:

- Is the explanation appropriate for the injury sustained in terms of mechanism, force or dating of the injury? OI is more likely when (a) the fracture site is consistent with the history but the force involved in the injury seems too minor to have caused the fracture; (b) fractures recur in a protected environment; and (c) when there are no external signs of abuse.
- Is there bruising in unusual areas, such as on the back, ears and genitalia, suggestive of NAI?
- Is there evidence of an underlying skeletal abnormality which has predisposed to the fracture, i.e. signs suggestive of OI, such as blue sclerae, dentinogenesis imperfecta, hypermobility, flat feet?
- Is there positive family history of multiple fractures? It is possible though that a child has a new mutation of OI.
- What is the age of the patient? NAI is more common in younger children.

- Is there low BMD suggestive of osteoporosis? DXA scan needs to be performed in children older than 5 years.

In case of suspicion of NAI, a full skeletal survey needs to be performed.

Radiologic signs can assist in the differential diagnosis (**Figure 7.2**) [12].

- *Radiologic signs suggestive of OI*: Multiple Wormian bones, osteopenia on skeletal survey, long-bone deformities, mid-shaft fractures, multiple thoracolumbar compression fractures.
- *Radiologic signs suggestive of NAI*: Symmetric rib fractures, especially when they are posterior, metaphyseal fractures in children <1 year old, complex skull fractures, spinous process fractures, scapular and sternal fractures.

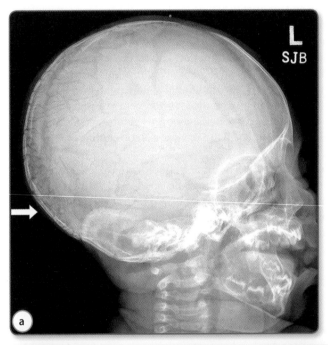

**Figure 7.2** (a) Plain x-ray and (b) CT images showing multiple Wormian bones in a child with osteogenesis imperfecta (from personal files of Dr Sakka).

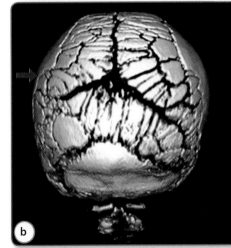
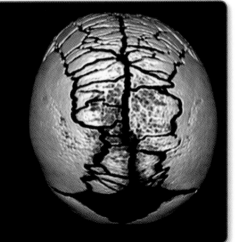

All the above factors need to be taken into account when investigating for NAI. Nowadays, with the increased introduction of genetics to clinical practice, diagnosis can be facilitated by targeted genetic panels looking for OI genes.

## Secondary osteoporosis

Some of the most common causes of secondary paediatric osteoporosis will be presented in order to increase awareness and prompt for early recognition.

### Cerebral palsy and other immobility-induced osteoporosis

The Mechanostat theory, initially proposed by Frost [13], explains how development of bone strength in childhood is driven by mechanical loads. Loss of these loads leads to loss of bone tissue strain and results in reductions in bone mass and in some cases disuse osteoporosis. Cerebral palsy (CP) is the most common cause of immobility, but any child that is wheelchair-bound is at risk of developing osteoporosis and subsequent fractures. The most frequent fracture sites are the distal femur and proximal tibia. The prevalence of fractures in CP ranges between 6 and 50% [14]. Prophylactic treatment with bisphosphonates is not justified, but they should be offered in case of fractures [15].

### Leukaemia

Osteoporotic fractures are a significant cause of morbidity in acute lymphoblastic leukaemia (ALL). Results from the STeroid-associated Osteoporosis in the Paediatric Population (STOPP) study that followed 186 children with leukaemia for 6 years since diagnosis revealed a cumulative fracture incidence of 32.5% for VFs and 23% for non-VF, while 39% of children were asymptomatic. The incidence of fractures was significantly related to baseline VF, glucocorticoid (GC) dose, and baseline LS BMD Z-score. Most of these fractures had re-shaped with treatment within the 6 years follow-up period, but 22.7% had persistent vertebral deformity, mostly older children and those with more severe collapse [16]. These results suggest that children diagnosed with leukaemia should be screened with DXA scan and lateral spine images at diagnosis and should be followed with repeated assessments during treatment or with symptoms of back pain.

### Intestinal failure and inflammatory bowel disease

A systematic review found a low bone-mineral mass or density in up to 45% of children with intestinal failure (IF) needing parenteral nutrition (PN), supporting the necessity of bone assessment in the follow-up of children with IF. Specifically, patients with motility disorders (congenital intestinal pseudo-obstruction, long-segment Hirschsprung's disease, and total or near-total aganglionosis) and congenital or early-onset enteropathies were at higher risk of developing metabolic bone disease (MBD). This could be the consequence of insufficiency of micro- and macronutrients in a malnourished patient [17]. This review emphasised the importance of long-term monitoring of children with PN, even after cessation of PN. The most recent guidelines on paediatric PN suggest measurement of BMD with DXA on a 2–3 yearly basis or annually if previously abnormal [18].

In IBD, mainly Crohn disease (CD), skeletal health can be affected due to the direct effects of chronic inflammation, prolonged use of GC, poor nutrition, delayed puberty and low muscle mass [19,20]. Inflammatory cytokines reduce bone formation and increase bone resorption. Also, osteotoxic medications such as GCs further deteriorate bone mineral density and bone structure. Transiliac biopsies in children with IBD showed thin cortices and reduced bone formation rates on trabecular surfaces consistent with a low bone turnover rate [21]. A systematic review in IBD and osteoporosis in children reported a prevalence of osteoporosis between 4 and 9% in studies including both CD and ulcerative colitis (UC) patients; 2–9% in studies including UC patients, and 7–15% in studies including CD patients. CD diagnosis, lower body mass index (BMI), and lower body weight were risk factors associated with osteoporosis or low BMD [22]. Therefore, monitoring of these children with DXA scans and spine X-rays along with evaluation for back pain is recommended.

## Delayed or suspended puberty

Albright recognised the significance of sex steroids on skeletal maturation and preservation from the early 40s. The production of sex steroids at the start of puberty is clearly linked with an increase of bone mineral acquisition during this period [23,24]. Oestrogens bind with oestrogen receptor to promote the expression of osteoprotegerin (OPG), and to suppress the action of nuclear factor-κβ ligand (RANKL), thus inhibiting osteoclast formation and bone resorptive activity. They can also increase osteogenesis. The net effects of oestrogen deficiency are increased bone turnover and enhanced bone resorption, which result in osteoporosis [25]. Testosterone converts into oestrogens in the tissues, and both are present in men and women in different amounts. Deprivation of sex steroids due to delayed or suspended puberty in conditions such as Turner's syndrome, anorexia nervosa, primary ovarian failure, ovarian or testicular failure as a result of cancer treatment, long-term high-dose steroid use can negatively affect bone mineral density and maximum bone mass acquisition. Therefore, pubertal status and hormonal levels should be assessed in patients at risk and timely supplementation with oestrogens or testosterone should be offered in order to protect their bones.

## Glucocorticoid use

Glucocorticoids are the most widely used anti-inflammatory drug around the world. However, one of the most severe adverse effects is osteoporosis. They decrease the proliferation of osteogenic precursors and suppress of osteoblasts, reducing bone formation. They also increase RANKL/OPG ratio which promotes bone resorption by enhancing the maturation and activation of osteoclasts. As a result, bone integrity is reduced and the risk of fracture is increased [25]. The Canadian STOPP study followed large numbers of children on steroids for systemic illnesses and along with other studies, gave us a lot of information on the natural history of systemic illness osteoporosis and the monitoring strategies for the early identification of fragility fractures in children with secondary osteoporosis. It is important that all children on high-dose chronic steroid use are monitored for osteoporosis.

Predictors of incident vertebral fracture in GC use [26] are:

- Signs of excess GC exposure
- Declines in LS BMD Z-score in first 6 months of treatment
- Increased in BMI
- Worsening of disease control

## Rheumatic disorders

Rheumatic disorders in children include juvenile dermatomyositis, juvenile idiopathic arthritis (JIA), systemic lupus erythematosus, systemic vasculitis, and other. The mainstay of treatment includes high-dose corticosteroids, especially at diagnosis and during relapses. The STOPP consortium monitored 136 children with GC-treated rheumatoid conditions and revealed a 6-year cumulative fracture incidence of 16.3% for VF and 10.1% for non-VF. 63% of these fractures occurred in the first 2 years from diagnosis, which is the period of maximum GC exposure. Fortunately, 84% had complete vertebral body reshaping, but vertebral deformity persisted in the rest [27]. Therefore, children with back pain or poorly controlled underlying disease and >3 months on high-dose steroids or chronic reduced mobility should undergo bone-health monitoring, including spine imaging [26].

## Duchenne muscular dystrophy

In Duchenne muscular dystrophy (DMD) osteoporosis is precipitated by the combination of three risk factors: (a) chronic use of high-dose steroids, (b) absence of the anabolic effect of testosterone on bones due to delayed puberty, which is also a result of steroid use, and (c) immobilisation. The UK NorthStar database included data from 832 boys with DMD from 23 centres. Fracture incidence rate was at least four times higher than in healthy boys. There was a 50% probability of first fracture by the age of 11 years and it increased with duration of treatment and age. Boys treated with daily deflazacort had the highest fracture incidence rate, while the risk was smaller with intermittent use of steroids [28]. Boys with DMD experience premature, permanent loss of ambulation following a long-bone fracture [29]. Also, if vertebral fractures are left untreated, they can lead to a 'vertebral fracture cascade' which causes significant morbidity and affects their quality of life [30]. Therefore, DMD Care Considerations Working Group published guidance in 2018 advising for early monitoring of bone health with DXA and either spinal X-ray or VFA and treatment with bisphosphonates when indicated [31].

# WHAT IS THE TREATMENT OF PAEDIATRIC OSTEOPOROSIS?

The objective of treatment of osteoporosis in children is to maximise bone strength, to decrease the risk of fractures, and to re-shape vertebral fractures. Underlying risk factors, such as primary osteoporosis condition, duration of corticosteroid use, severity of disease-causing secondary osteoporosis, possibility of automatic recovery should also be taken into account and may alter our decision on treatment. Furthermore, treatment needs to start before attainment of adult height in order to increase chances of vertebral body reshaping. It is suggested that children with a suspicion or diagnosis of primary or secondary osteoporosis should be referred to a specialist with experience in managing these conditions.

## How to reduce the risk for osteoporosis?

- Reduction of sedentary life and increase in physical activity
- Achievement of optimal levels of Vitamin D by:
  - More outdoor time and access to direct sunlight. Inadequate serum Vitamin D is associated with secondary hyperparathyroidism, increased bone turnover, accelerated bone loss, and increased fracture risk [32].
  - Vitamin D supplementation, especially in at-risk groups

- Optimal intake of calcium, protein and calories
- Suppression of chronic inflammation
- Reduction of steroid use when possible and use of alternative steroid-sparing regimens
- Pubertal induction or sex steroid supplementation of children with delayed or suspended puberty
- Early recognition of conditions like anorexia nervosa that can affect both nutritional intake, but also suppresses endogenous sex steroid production.

When all other measures have failed to prevent or treat osteoporotic fractures, the use of bisphosphonates should be considered. Bisphosphonates are pyrophosphate-derived medications that inhibit osteoclastic function. They are used on an off-label basis and are the pharmacologic agent with the longest experience in the treatment of paediatric osteoporosis. Pamidronate has been used most extensively but has been now replaced in most centres by the most potent bisphosphonate zoledronic acid (ZA), because it can be infused more rapidly and less frequently. The duration of treatment depends on the underlying condition. Our decision to treat should also be affected by the potential of vertebral fractures to reshape without treatment and the persistence or not of risk factors [15,33].

## CONCLUSION

Paediatric osteoporosis is an under-recognised condition that can lead to long bone and vertebral fractures and increased morbidity in later life. Paediatricians and general practitioners, as well as specialists dealing with children with chronic conditions that could be related with reduced bone density and adverse effects on bones, should be able to recognise risk factors and monitor for osteoporosis. Advice should be given on how to change lifestyle and diet, but also how to alter predisposing factors for osteoporosis. Early recognition and referral to specialists that could offer more specialised treatment, such as bisphosphonates, can alter the course of the disease and improve the quality of life of these patients.

## REFERENCES

1.  Bishop N, Arundel P, Clark E et al. Fracture prediction and the definition of osteoporosis in children and adolescents: The ISCD 2013 Pediatric Official Positions. J Clin Densitom 2014; 17:275–280
2.  Genant HK, Wu CY, van Kuijk C, Nevitt MC. Vertebral fracture assessment using a semiquantitative technique. J Bone Miner Res 1993; 8:1137–1148.
3.  Ward LM, Weber DR, Munns CF, Hogler W, Zemel BS. A Contemporary View of the Definition and Diagnosis of Osteoporosis in Children and Adolescents. J Clin Endocrinol Metab 2020; 105:e2088-e2097.
4.  Weber DR, Boyce A, Gordon C, et al. The Utility of DXA Assessment at the Forearm, Proximal Femur, and Lateral Distal Femur, and Vertebral Fracture Assessment in the Pediatric Population: 2019 ISCD Official Position. J Clin Densitom 2019; 22:567–589.
5.  Zemel BS, Leonard MB, Kelly A, et al. Height adjustment in assessing dual energy x-ray absorptiometry measurements of bone mass and density in children. J Clin Endocrinol Metab 2010; 95:1265–1273.
6.  Crabtree NJ, Shaw NJ, Bishop NJ, et al. Amalgamated Reference Data for Size-Adjusted Bone Densitometry Measurements in 3598 Children and Young Adults-the ALPHABET Study. J Bone Miner Res 2017; 32:172–180.
7.  Trejo P, Rauch F. Osteogenesis imperfecta in children and adolescents-new developments in diagnosis and treatment. Osteoporosis international 2016; 27:3427–3437.

8.   Sillence DO, Senn A, Danks DM. Genetic heterogeneity in osteogenesis imperfecta. Journal of medical genetics 1979; 16:101–116.

9.   Thomas IH, DiMeglio LA. Advances in the Classification and Treatment of Osteogenesis Imperfecta. Current osteoporosis reports 2016; 14:1–9.

10.  Lorenc, RS. Idiopathic Juvenile Osteoporosis. Calcif Tissue Int 2002; 70:395–397.

11.  Chapman S, Hall CM. Non-accidental injury or brittle bones. Pediatric Radiology 1997; 27:106–110.

12.  Pereira EM. Clinical perspectives on osteogenesis imperfecta versus non-accidental injury. Am J Med Genet C Semin Med Genet 2015; 169:302–306.

13.  Frost HM. Bone "mass" and the "mechanostat": a proposal. The Anatomical record 1987; 219:1–9.

14.  Presedo A, Dabney KW, Miller F. Fractures in patients with cerebral palsy. J Pediatr Orthop 2007; 27:147–153.

15.  Simm PJ, Biggin A, Zacharin MR, et al. Consensus guidelines on the use of bisphosphonate therapy in children and adolescents. J Paediatr Child Health 2018; 54:223–233.

16.  Ward LM, Ma J, Lang B et al; Steroid-Associated Osteoporosis in the Pediatric Population (STOPP) Consortium. Bone Morbidity and Recovery in Children With Acute Lymphoblastic Leukemia: Results of a Six-Year Prospective Cohort Study. J Bone Miner Res 2018; 33:1435–1443.

17.  Gatti S, Quattrini S, Palpacelli A, Catassi GN, Lionetti ME, Catassi C. Metabolic Bone Disease in Children with Intestinal Failure and Long-Term Parenteral Nutrition: A Systematic Review Nutrients 2022;14:995.

18.  Hill S, Ksiazyk J, Prell C, Tabbers M, ESPGHAN/ESPEN/ESPR/CSPEN Working Group on Pediatric Parenteral Nutrition. ESPGHAN/ESPEN/ESPR/CSPEN guidelines on pediatric parenteral nutrition: Home parenteral nutrition. Clin Nutr 2018; 37:2401–2408.

19.  Wong SC, Catto-Smith AG, Zacharin M. Pathological fractures in paediatric patients with inflammatory bowel disease. Eur J Pediatr 2014; 173:141–151.

20.  Pappa H, Thayu M, Sylvester F, Leonard M, Zemel B, Gordon C. Skeletal health of children and adolescents with inflammatory bowel disease. J Pediatr Gastroenterol Nutr 2011; 53:11–25.

21.  Ward LM, Rauch F, Matzinger MA, Benchimol EI, Boland M, Mack DR. Iliac bone histomorphometry in children with newly diagnosed inflammatory bowel disease. Osteoporos Int 2010; 21:331–337.

22.  Kärnsund S, Lo B, Bendtsen F, Holm J, Burisch J. Systematic review of the prevalence and development of osteoporosis or low bone mineral density and its risk factors in patients with inflammatory bowel disease. World J Gastroenterol 2020; 26:5362–5374.

23.  Seeman E. From density to structure: growing up and growing old on the surfaces of bone. J Bone Miner Res 1997; 12:509–521

24.  Vandewalle S, Taes Y, Fiers T, et al. Associations of sex steroids with bone maturation, bone mineral density, bone geometry, and body composition: a cross-sectional study in healthy male adolescents. J Clin Endocrinol Metab 2014; 99:E1272–E1282.

25.  Cheng CH, Chen LR, Chen KH. Osteoporosis Due to Hormone Imbalance: An Overview of the Effects of Estrogen Deficiency and Glucocorticoid Overuse on Bone Turnover. Int J Mol Sci 2022; 23:1376.

26.  Ward LM. Part I: Which Child with a Chronic Disease Needs Bone Health Monitoring? Curr Osteoporos Rep. 2021; 19:278–288.

27.  Ward LM, Ma J, Robinson ME, et al. Osteoporotic Fractures and Vertebral Body Reshaping in Children With Glucocorticoid-treated Rheumatic Disorders. J Clin Endocrinol Metab 2021; 106:e5195–e5207.

28.  Joseph S, Wang C, Bushby K, et al; UK NorthStar Clinical Network. Fractures and Linear Growth in a Nationwide Cohort of Boys With Duchenne Muscular Dystrophy With and Without Glucocorticoid Treatment: Results From the UK NorthStar Database. JAMA Neurol 2019; 76:701–709.

29.  Ma J, McMillan HJ, Karaguzel G, et al. The time to and determinants of first fractures in boys with Duchenne muscular dystrophy. Osteoporos Int 2017; 28:597–608.

30.  Christiansen BA, Bouxsein ML. Biomechanics of vertebral fractures and the vertebral fracture cascade. Current osteoporosis reports 2010; 8:198–204.

31.  Birnkrant DJ, Bushby K, Bann CM, et al. Diagnosis and management of Duchenne muscular dystrophy, part 2: respiratory, cardiac, bone health, and orthopaedic management. Lancet Neurol 2018; 17:347–361.

32. Munns CF, Shaw N, Kiely M, et al. Global Consensus Recommendations on Prevention and Management of Nutritional Rickets. Horm Res Paediatr 2016; 85:83–106.

33. Ward LM. Part 2: When Should Bisphosphonates Be Used in Children with Chronic Illness Osteoporosis? Curr Osteoporos Rep 2021; 19:289–297.

# Chapter 8

## Advances in paediatric surgery

*Vanessa Coles, I Yardley*

## INTRODUCTION

Paediatric surgery remains an anomaly among surgical specialities, being the only one defined by the age of the patient rather than their presenting condition. While some areas have been incorporated into other surgical specialities, most obviously paediatric cardiac surgery, paediatric neurosurgery and paediatric orthopaedics; paediatric general surgery still encompasses a broad range of conditions and presentations including abdominal surgery, thoracic surgery, oncological surgery, and urology. The general paediatric surgeon can expect to encounter and care for patients ranging from the most premature new-born infant to patients in young adulthood. In this chapter, we explore the recent advances this unique speciality has seen and touch on what the future may hold.

Due to the array of presentations the speciality encompasses and the rarity of many of the conditions treated, paediatric surgery has been undergoing a process of sub-specialisation. The rationale for this being the evidence of volume-outcome relationships and improved outcomes in adult surgical conditions following sub-specialisation [1]. The most obvious sub-division within the specialty is between 'Paediatric General Surgery' and 'Paediatric Urology'; however, other conditions are also commonly concentrated into fewer hands, for example, in most paediatric surgical units, not every surgeon would undertake major oncological resections. In larger units it is possible to extend the process of sub-specialisation further, for example, to upper and lower gastro-intestinal surgery. This is more challenging in smaller units, especially when the provision of emergency cover is considered, meaning that, for many, paediatric surgeries remains a very general surgical practice. It should be noted that the evidence for improved outcomes in paediatric surgery following sub-specialisation is limited and we remain a significant way off sub-specialisation being formally recognised across the board in paediatric surgery.

An extension of the discussion of whether to formalise sub-specialisation in paediatric surgery is the concept of centralisation for particularly rare conditions. Nominating selected centres to take all cases in that country of a certain condition will lead to a higher volume treated by a dedicated team, rather than the current system of each centre

**Vanessa Coles** MRCS, Jenny Lind Children's Hospital, Norwich, UK
Email: vanessa.coles2@nhs.net

**Iain Yardley** FRCS, Evelina London Children's Hospital, London, UK
Email: Iain.yardley@gstt.nhs.uk

seeing an average of fewer than one or two cases a year. This model has been successfully implemented in the United Kingdom (UK) for both Biliary Atresia and Bladder Exstrophy [2]. Discussions are ongoing as to which other conditions may benefit from centralisation, with Oesophageal Atresia with Tracheo-oesphageal Fistula (OA-TOF), particularly 'long-gap' variants, and congenital diaphragmatic hernia (CDH) being two conditions currently under scrutiny [3].

## ADVANCES IN RESEARCH

It is widely acknowledged that high-quality research helps to shape, improve and advance good surgical practice. However, conducting definitive trials, especially randomised control trials can be difficult in children. Firstly, the rarity of many conditions requires lengthy, multi-centre and therefore costly studies to be carried out. Additionally, research in children creates additional complexity surrounding the ethics of and consent for research [4–6].

Specialist paediatric surgical journals remain dominated by single-centre, usually retrospective, case-based studies. These have their place, especially where sub-specialisation has created larger volume series and supported research alongside clinical care, however, there has been a gradual shift in mentality in the paediatric surgical community that collaboration, both nationally and internationally, is key to advance academia in paediatric surgery [5].

With this shift in focus towards collaborative work, several significant projects have been completed. One example is the British Association of Paediatric Surgeons Congenital Anomalies Surveillance System (BAPS-CASS). BAPS-CASS was a system that engaged surgeons across the UK to report each case of a given neonatal index condition they managed over the course of a 12-month period, thereby building up a cohort prospectively [7]. Conditions covered included oesophageal atresia, gastroschisis, necrotising enterocolitis (NEC) and meconium ileus. The surveillance system has now closed, but relatively large, prospective studies, including those that examine longer term outcomes, continue to be published from the cohorts collected, demonstrating the potential that large collaborative endeavours have [8,9].

Increasingly, randomised controlled trials (RCTs) are being carried out in paediatric surgery. These have covered topics as diverse as NEC and appendicitis [10,11]. These are commonly multi-centre and long term, making securing funding for the studies challenging.

## ADVANCES IN CLINICAL ASPECTS

The greatest improvements in patient outcomes in paediatric surgery are not down to great advances in surgical technique, but rather to a huge improvement in the surrounding medical care of paediatric surgical patients. This is most clearly seen in neonatal surgery with the huge progress that has occurred in neonatal intensive care medicine. Stepwise advances in our understanding of the role of interventions such as maternal steroids, inhaled surfactant, inhaled nitric oxide (iNO) and high-frequency oscillation have allowed survival at progressively lower gestational ages [12]. The development in the 1960s of appropriately sized catheters and tailored parenteral nutrition (PN) solutions for extremely premature infants has led to huge improvements in nutrition and growth [13]. This has had a direct impact on morbidity and mortality outcomes in those infants who undergo surgery for conditions where the gut cannot be used for nutrition such as necrotising enterocolitis and gastroschisis [13,14].

There have been significant refinements in the understanding and management of congenital abnormalities on the neonatal and paediatric intensive care units. The CDH is a good example. It is now well established that a period of stabilisation for patients with CDH is vital prior to any attempt at surgical correction [15,16]. The practice of 'gentle ventilation' and permissive hypercapnia has greatly reduced the incidence of barotrauma to the lung and improved the outcomes of this patient cohort [17,18]. We are continuing to define the role of adjuncts such as iNO and extra-corporal membrane oxygenation (ECMO).

There has been a particularly remarkable rise in the expected survival of patients born with OA-TOF within the course of a single lifetime. At the time of the first successful repair in 1948 survival was around 30%, it is now well above 90% in most centres with the majority of mortality burden coming from associated conditions such as congenital cardiac lesions [13,19]. While surgical technique has undoubtedly improved in this time, the improved survival is largely due to the improvements in neonatal care discussed above, including management of medical co-morbidities, improved ventilation methods, and the availability of tailored PN.

Away from the neonatal unit, there have been other advances in and changes to clinical care. In the general paediatric population, appendicitis is the most common abdominal emergency. Over the years there has been a shift from the traditional open appendicectomy towards a more minimally invasive approach as paediatric surgeons have caught up with their adult counterparts. Advances to laparoscopic equipment, increased experience of laparoscopy among paediatric surgeons and increasing evidence of the benefits has led to the majority of paediatric patients now undergoing a laparoscopic rather than open appendicectomy [20]. The management of acute appendicitis in children is currently under question, with the assumption that appendicectomy is the optimal management being challenged. The suggestion that simple appendicitis is best treated non-operatively has been advanced over recent years, with several centres publishing their positive experiences [21]. The coronavirus disease 2019 (COVID-19) pandemic gave impetus to this agenda as the availability of emergency surgery was limited and children were treated pragmatically with antibiotics alone [22]. In 2021, a successful feasibility trial was completed in the UK, randomising patients with appendicitis to operative or non-operative management (CONTRACT) and the main trial is due to start soon [11]. If conclusive, the findings of this study could radically alter the approach taken to childhood appendicitis.

## ADVANCES IN SURGICAL TECHNIQUES

Advances in surgical techniques and equipment tend to be slower in paediatric surgery than in adult surgery. This is for a variety of reasons, but the smaller commercial market created by varied patient size and rare pathology in paediatric surgery plays a significant part as it inhibits industry investment. For example, there was an initial hesitation from paediatric surgeons to take up minimally invasive surgery (MIS) when it was first introduced due to concerns that instruments were not appropriately sized for the majority of their patients [20]. Since then, improvements in the equipment available, in particular the introduction of shorter, 3 mm diameter laparoscopic instruments, have allowed paediatric laparoscopic and thoracoscopic surgery to advance significantly.

Common conditions such as appendicitis and pyloric stenosis are now routinely treated laparoscopically with consistently lower wound infections and reduced length of hospital stay [23,24]. Even management of inguinal hernias has moved towards a minimally invasive approach, with this being the approach of choice for many surgeons, particularly in the infant patient cohort. Laparoscopy provides the advantage of diagnosing and treating both the symptomatic and a latent contralateral hernia under one anaesthetic with comparable recurrence rates to the open approach [25]. The drive to expand the application of MIS continues including in neonatal cases such as CDH and OA-TOF [20].

There have also been moves to advance the concept of MIS ever further, in several ways. One is the use of single-incision laparoscopy in children, with appendicitis being the initial area of focus for this novel technique with some early promising results [26,27]. Robotic or, more accurately, robot-assisted surgery, is a further advance in the concept of MIS. A few centres have demonstrated the feasibility of robotic surgery in a paediatric patient cohort, but there remain barriers to cross in terms of appropriately sized instruments and a consensus on which patients would benefit most from this technique [28,29] before this is likely to become widespread, especially when the high financial cost, both in capital and operating expenditure are taken into account. Lastly, advanced endoscopic procedures as an alternative to surgical approaches are becoming more established in adult surgical practice and this is slowly transferring across to paediatric patients as well. Probably the most established advance in endoscopy in paediatric surgery so far is the use of per-oral endoscopic myotomy (POEM) for achalasia. A systematic review and meta-analysis in 2019 showed the promise of this technique; however further research, ideally as an RCT, is needed before confirming any preference of POEM over more established techniques [30].

There are several challenges faced when trying to implement MIS in the paediatric population. Case numbers in individual centres for the rarest congenital abnormalities remain low, making gaining training and experience challenging. There is also a lack of clear evidence of patient benefit from MIS and the challenge of operating in such a tiny space as found in a neonate, means that compromises in surgical accuracy are inevitable and this creates reluctance on the part of many surgeons to adopt MIS techniques. It seems likely that as instrument technology evolves and improves these compromises will be reduced, evidence of benefit will emerge, and the use of MIS is likely to expand [20].

## ADVANCES IN FETAL SURGERY

Fetal surgery involves operating on a fetus in utero. This can be conducted via several approaches, including open and MIS (hysteroscopic) surgery. There have been huge advances in recent years, both with the techniques and equipment available but also with the number of conditions that can successfully be treated [31], babies diagnosed antenatally with previously fatal conditions can now be given a chance for survival. Careful consideration of the risks and benefits of intervention and subsequent patient selection remains paramount; however, as fetal surgery is not without significant risk both to the fetus and the mother. Any centre offering fetal surgery must be able to fully counsel the parents and be equipped and prepared for potential preterm labour [32].

One of the first conditions to benefit from intra-uterine intervention was twin-to-twin transfusion syndrome (TTTS). In 2004, the RCT demonstrated a higher rate of survival in twins who underwent intra-uterine endoscopic laser ablation of aberrant placental vessels, compared to those who underwent serial amnioreduction therapy [33]. Fetal laser ablation has now become the primary treatment for TTTS and its success has sparked further advances in other fetal anomalies.

Probably the best evidenced fetal surgical intervention is the intra-uterine closure of myelomeningocele (MMC). This is the most common severe neural tube defect seen and can be easily detected at the 20-week fetal scan. Infants affected suffer from hydrocephalus and cognitive impairment along with varying degrees of lower limb paralysis and incontinence. Following successful lamb models in 1995, a major RCT in America demonstrated dramatically improved infantile neurological outcomes, albeit at the expense of increased rates of premature birth and maternal morbidity [34,35]. Current work is on developing and refining surgical techniques, including MIS, to maintain the benefits of this fetal surgery and minimise the drawbacks [35].

Congenital diaphragmatic hernia is another condition where fetal intervention has been attempted. The CDH is characterised by herniation of abdominal contents into the thoracic cavity leading to significant lung hypoplasia and pulmonary hypertension. Extrapolating from the finding of abnormally large lungs in infants with laryngeal atresia, fetal tracheal occlusion has been deployed to improve lung growth [36]. Initially, tracheal clipping in utero was tried, which then progressed to internal occlusion of the trachea via a balloon, known as 'Fetoscopic Endoluminal Tracheal Occlusion (FETO)' [36]. Earlier this year the results of the Tracheal Occlusion to Accelerate Lung Growth (TOTAL) trial were published with promising results. The TOTAL-trial was a randomised control trial that looked at both moderate and severe left-sided CDHs and the outcomes when FETO was performed [37,38]. Although in the moderate group there was no benefit seen with FETO over expectant care when FETO was performed at 30–32 weeks, there was a significant benefit seen in the severe group [37,38].

A good example of the limitations of fetal surgery is lower urinary tract obstruction. This can occur due to a variety of reasons, posterior urethral valves being the most common. It can lead to renal dysplasia, oligohydramnios and pulmonary hypoplasia, it seems intuitive that bypassing the obstruction with a vesico-amniotic shunt should obviate these risks and allow normal fetal development and this technique was first described over 40 years ago [39]. Unfortunately, no clear benefit has been demonstrated from this technique and the PLUTO (Percutaneous vesico-amniotic shunting for fetal Lower Urinary Tract Obstruction) RCT failed to recruit sufficient numbers of patients and was abandoned unfinished, leaving the role of vesico-amniotic shunting unclear [40].

## CONCLUSION

In this chapter, we have highlighted just a few of the advances and changes currently being seen in paediatric surgery. As a surgical speciality that is still relatively young, it is one on an exciting path of discovery and improvements to the care of infants and children who require surgical intervention both before and after birth. These developments are likely to continue to be due to a combination of medical advances, technological refinements and research collaborations.

# REFERENCES

1.  Boddy AP, Williamson JM, Vipond MN. The effect of centralisation on the outcomes of oesophagogastric surgery – a fifteen year audit. Int J Surg 2012; 10:360-363.
2.  Durkin N, Davenport M. Centralization of Pediatric Surgical Procedures in the United Kingdom. Eur J Pediatr Surg 2017; 27:416–421.
3.  GIRFT. The GIRFT national report on paediatric surgery and urology. [Internet]. Viewed 29th April 2022. Available from https://www.gettingitrightfirsttime.co.uk/surgical-speciality/paediatric-surgery. (Last accessed 18th January 2023).
4.  Losty P. The Challenges of surgical research in children. BJS 2017; 104:1589–1590.
5.  Curry J, Reeves B, Stringer M. Randomized control trials in pediatric surgery: could we do better? J Pediatr Surg 2003; 38:556–559.
6.  Johnson P. Paediatric surgical research in the UK – Challenges and opportunities. Semin Pediatr Surg 2021; 30:151019.
7.  NPEU. British Association of Paediatric Surgeons Congenital Anomalies Surveillance System (BAPS-CASS). [Internet]. 2022. Available from https://www.npeu.ox.ac.uk/baps-cass. (Last accessed 18th January 2023).
8.  Bethell G, Long AM, Knight M, Hall N. Congenital duodenal obstruction in the UK: a population-based study. Arch Dis Child Fetal Neonatal Ed 2020; 105:178–183.
9.  Brownlee E, Wragg R, Robb A, et al. Current epidemiology and antenatal presentation of posterior urethral valves: Outcome of BAPS CASS National Audit. J Pediatr Surg 2019; 54:318–321.
10. Rees CM, Eaton S, Kiely EM, et al. Peritoneal drainage or laparotomy for neonatal bowel perforation? A randomised controlled trial. Ann Surg 2008; 248:44–51.
11. Hall NJ, Eaton S, Sherratt FC, et al. CONservative Treatment of Appendicitis in Children: a randomised controlled feasibility Trial (CONTRACT). Arch Dis Child 2021; 106:764–773.
12. Rennie J, Bokhari S. Recent advances in neonatology. Arch Dis Childhood – Fetal Neonat Ed 1999; 81:F1–F4.
13. Holland A, McBride C. Non-operative advances: what has happened in the last 50 years in paediatric surgery? J Paediatr Child Health 2015; 51:74–77.
14. Rowe M, Rowe S. The last fifty years of neonatal surgical management. Am J Surg 2000; 180:345–352.
15. Reiss I, Schaible T, van den Hout L, et al. Standardized postnatal management of infants with congenital diaphragmatic hernia in Europe: The CDH EURO Consortium consensus. Neonatology 2010; 98:354–364.
16. Moyer V, Moya F, Tibboel R, et al. Late versus early surgical correction for congenital diaphragmatic hernia in newborn infants. Cochrane Database Syst Rev 2002; 3:CD001695.
17. Wilson J, Lund D, Lillwhei C, Vacanti J. Congenital Diaphragmatic hernia – a tale of two cities: the Boston experience. J Pediatr Surg 1997; 32:401–405.
18. Sluiter I, van de Ven C, Wijnen R, Tibboel D. Congenital diaphragmatic hernia: still a moving target. Semin Fetal Neonatal Med 2011; 16:139–144.
19. Holland A, Fitzgerald D. Oesophageal atresia and trachea-oesophageal fistula: current management strategies and complications. Paediatr Respir Rev 2010; 11:100–106.
20. Blantnik J, Ponsky T. Advances in Minimally Invasive Surgery in Pediatrics. Curr Gastroenterol Reports 2010; 12:211–214.
21. Georgiou R, Eaton S, Stanton M, Pierro A, Hall N. Efficacy and Safety of Nonoperative Treatment for Acute Appendicitis: A Meta-analysis. Pediatrics 2017; 139:e20163003.
22. Bethell GS, Gosling T, Rees CM, Sutcliffe J, Hall NJ. CASCADE Study Collaborators and the RIFT Study Collaborators. Impact of the COVID-19 pandemic on management and outcomes of children with appendicitis: The Children with AppendicitiS during the CoronAvirus pandemic (CASCADE) study. J Pediatr Surg 2022; 57:380–385.
23. Sauerland S, Lefering R, Neugebauer E. Laparoscopic verses open surgery for suspected appendicitis. Cochrane Database Syst Rev 2004; 4:CD001546.
24. Markar SR, Blackburn S, Cobb R, et al. Laparoscopic versus open appendectomy in children with uncomplicated and complicated appendicitis. J Pediatr Surg 2004; 39:1680–1685.

25. Kantor N, Travis N, Wayne C, Nasr A. Laparoscopic versus open inguinal hernia repair in children: which is the true gold-standard? A systematic review and meta-analysis. Pedatr Surg Int 2019; 35:1013–1026.

26. Chow A, Aziz O, Purkayastha S, Darzi A, Paraskeva P. Single Incision Laparoscopic Surgery for Acute Appendicitis: Feasibility in Pediatric Patients. Diagn Ther Endosc 2010; 294958.

27. Ming YC, Yang W, Chen JC, Chang PY, Lai JY. Experience of single-incision laparoscopy in children. J Minim Access Surg 2016; 12:245–247.

28. Lima M, Thomas E, Si Salvo N, Gargano T, Ruggeri G. Paediatric surgery in the robotic era: early experience and comparative analysis. Pediatr Med Chir 2019; 41.

29. Cave J, Clarke S. Paediatric robotic surgery. Ann R Coll Surg Eng 2018; 100:18–21.

30. Lee Y, Brar K, Doumouras A, Hong D. Peroral endoscopic myotomy (POEM) for the treatment of pediatric achalasia: a systematic review and meta-analysis. Surg Endosc 2019; 33:1710–1720.

31. Sampat K, Losty P. Fetal Surgery. BJS 2021; 108:632–637.

32. Deprest J, Jani J, Lewi L, et al. Fetoscopic surgery: encouraged by clinical experience and boosted by instrument innovation. Semin Fetal Neonatal Med 2006; 11:398–412.

33. Senat MV, Deprest J, Boulvain M, et al. Endoscopic laser surgery versus serial amnioreduction for severe twin-to-twin transfusion syndrome. N Engl J Med 2004; 351:136–144.

34. Meuli M, Meuli-Simmen C, Hutchins GM, et al. In utero surgery rescues neurological function at birth in sheep with spina bifida. Nat Med 1995; 1:342–347.

35. Adzick NS, Thom EA, Spong CY, et al. A randomized trial of prenatal versus postnatal repair of myelomeningocele. N Engl J Med 2011; 364:993–1004.

36. Harrison MR, Adzick NS, Flake AW, et al. Correction of congenital diaphragmatic hernia in utero: VI. hard-earned lessons. J Pediatr Surg 1993; 28:1411–1418.

37. Deprest JA, Benachi A, Gratacos E, et al. Randomized Trial of Fetal Surgery for Moderate Left Diaphragmatic Hernia. N Engl J Med 2021; 385:119–129.

38. Deprest JA, Nicolaides KH, Benachi A, et al. Randomized Trial of Fetal Surgery for Severe Left Diaphragmatic Hernia. N Engl J Med 2021; 385:107–118.

39. Harrison MR, Golbus MS, Filly RA, et al. Fetal surgery for congenital hydronephrosis. N Engl J Med 1981; 306:591–593.

40. Morris RK, Malin GL, Quinlan-Jones E, et al. Percutaneous vesicoamniotic shunting versus conservative management for fetal lower urinary tract obstruction (PLUTO): a randomised trial. Lancet 2013; 382:1496–1506.

# Chapter 9

# Posterior urethral valves

*Garriboli Massimo, Paraboschi Irene*

## DEFINITION, EPIDEMIOLOGY, AND CLASSIFICATION

Posterior urethral valves (PUVs) are congenital obstructing membranous folds of the male posterior urethra [1].

With a reported incidence of 1 in 3,800 male births per annum, PUVs represent the most common cause of bladder outlet obstruction in male infants and end-stage renal failure (ESRF) in the paediatric population [2].

Improvements in antenatal screening and ultrasound technology have set a prenatal detection rate of 35–50% of cases [2,3], being fetal bladder distension (megacystis), bilateral hydroureteronephrosis, and oligo-anhydramnios highly suspected for PUV [3] (**Figure 9.1**).

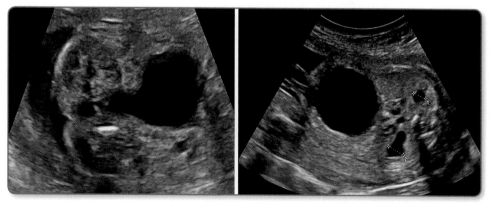

**Figure 9.1** Antenatal ultrasound scan of a male fetus with an enlarged, wall-thickened bladder associated with a dilated posterior urethra (Key-hole sign) and bilateral dilated kidneys (Evelina London Children's Hospital).

**Garriboli Massimo** MD FRCS(Eng) FEAPU FEBPS, Paediatric Nephro-Urology, Evelina London Children's Hospital, Guy's and St Thomas' NHS, Foundation Trust, London, UK
Email: massimo.garriboli@gstt.nhs.uk

**Paraboschi Irene** MD, Department of Paediatric Urology, Fondazione IRCCS Ca' Granda Ospedale Maggiore Policlinico Milano, Italia
Email: irene.paraboschi@hotmail.com

Despite recent progress in prenatal assessment and postnatal management, PUVs still represent one of the greatest challenges for paediatric urologists and paediatric nephrologists, with a quarter of children progressing to bladder decompensation and ESRF [4,5].

In 1919, Young et al [6] proposed the first systematic classification for PUV. Three main PUV types were identified:

1. Type 1 PUVs (accounting for 90–95% of all cases) are leaflets that extend inferiorly from the verumontanum towards the membranous urethra.
2. Type 2 PUVs (the rarest) are non-obstructing mucosal folds that extend from the verumontanum up towards the internal sphincter.
3. Type 3 PUVs (accounting for 5–10% of all cases) are concentric diaphragms that resemble a stricture and do not show any relationship with the verumontanum.

More recently, Dewan et al [7] suggested that the types 1 and 3 valves of Young's classification could, in fact, represent the same entity and described two main forms of congenital urethral obstructions, namely congenitally obstructing posterior urethral membrane (COPUM) and Cobb's collar. While COPUM was described as an oblique membrane intimately associated with the distal verumontanum, Cobb's collar was defined as a congenital urethral stricture located distally to the external urethral sphincter, showing no relationship with the verumontanum [8].

## EMBRYOLOGY

Although scientific observations and methodical investigations have spanned almost 200 years, there remains a lack of absolute certainty in understanding the origin of PUV.

The development of the male urethra starts during the 6th week of gestation with the urogenital sinus cavity extending onto the surface of the genital tubercle (**Figure 9.2**). This endodermal-derived groove later becomes a solid plate of cells that finally tabularise in a proximal-to-distal way to form the penile urethra, which completes its development at the 14th week of gestation [8].

The male urethra is traditionally divided into four distinct parts, each with its own anatomical classification, embryological origin, and histological cell type: proximally, the prostatic and the membranous urethra derive from the urogenital sinus and are composed of transitional epithelium, while, distally, the bulbar and the pendulous urethra derive from the genital tubercle and are lined with transitional and squamous epithelium [8].

In 1870, Tolmatschew first described PUV as 'overgrowths of the normally present anatomical folds and ridges in the urethra' [9].

Thirty years later, Bazy hypothesised that PUVs derive from the persistence of the urogenital membrane dividing the anterior from the posterior urethra [10], while Wilckens described PUV as remnants of the cloacal membrane, suggesting a stop in the embryological development as the underlying cause [11].

All these theories were based on post-mortem studies only. In this context, Lowsley was the first author to base his theory on PUV development on microscopic examination [12]. In his study, he noted that the PUVs were mainly made of dense connective tissue and smooth muscle fibres and suggested anomalies in the Wolffian or Müllerian ducts origin as the underlying cause for their origin.

Despite his method of dissecting was subsequently criticised, his studies marked the beginning of a more methodical and accurate way for investigating PUV origin.

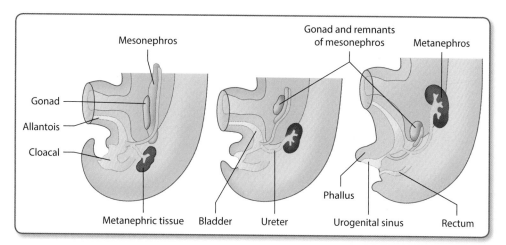

**Figure 9.2** Main steps of the development of the urinary tract.

Despite all the above-mentioned reports provided invaluable information for understanding the origin of PUV, their precise aetiology remains not fully defined. New reconstructive imaging modalities are therefore warranted to pinpoint the elusive embryology of PUV.

## AETIOLOGY

Posterior urethral valves seem to be a sporadic condition driven by a combination of genetic and environmental factors. Familial cases have been reported in the literature [13] together with a disproportionate incidence in African-American children and in boys affected by trisomy 21 [14] and Prune–Belly syndrome [15], however, PUVs usually occur in isolation and without other systems involved outside the urogenital tract.

## DIAGNOSIS

Nowadays, with the widespread use of prenatal screening, the most typical presentation for PUV is the antenatal finding of a thick-walled and dilated bladder associated with bilateral hydronephrosis, with subsequent diagnosis confirmed following birth [4].

Posterior urethral valves that are not suspected prenatally, usually present after birth with findings such as poor urinary stream, recurrent urinary tract infections (UTIs), and weight faltering [15].

In 23% of cases, PUVs are diagnosed in children older than 1 year of age because of urinary symptoms such as day- or night-time wetting, febrile UTIs, dribbling, urinary retention, or persistent haematuria [2,15].

Therefore, underlying structural problems should always be considered for male infants and children complaining of persistent lower urinary tract symptoms [15,16].

Although bladder and renal ultrasonography play a pivotal role in the initial screening of a child with suspected PUV, a micturating cystourethrogram (MCUG) is the most accurate radiological test used to identify a congenital infra-vesical obstruction [15,16] (**Figure 9.3**).

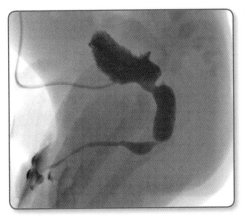

**Figure 9.3** Postnatal micturating cystourethrogram of a male patient showing a filling defect in the posterior urethra compatible with the diagnosis of posterior urethral valves (PUV) (Evelina London Children's Hospital).

In cases of PUV, highly specific radiological signs are a trabeculated bladder associated with a dilated posterior urethra. A secondary vesicoureteral reflux (VUR) is present in up to 50% of PUV cases [15,16]. A cystourethroscopy under general anaesthesia is, however, considered the gold standard for completing the diagnostic assessment, particularly in case the MCUG cannot provide a definitive diagnosis, often due to presence of artefacts related to the contraction of the striated external sphincter or when the quality of the radiograms is not ideal.

## INITIAL SURGICAL MANAGEMENT

In 35% of cases, PUVs are suspected *in utero* due to the detection of a fetal megacystis [2]. Children prenatally diagnosed with fetal megacystis carry a substantial risk of perinatal mortality and long-term morbidity [3]. The underlying bladder outlet obstruction can lead to high bladder pressure, bilateral kidney parenchymal compression and reduction of amniotic fluid (oligohydramnios), resulting in severe pulmonary hypoplasia and perinatal death in 35–55% of cases [17,18] and ESRF in 24–40% of survivors [3,17].

Therefore, in selected cases, fetal surgery such as vesicoamniotic shunting (VAS) or laser valve ablation has been recommended as rescue therapies to bypass the obstruction and attenuate the secondary structural complications [19].

The results of a randomised controlled trial investigating the effectiveness of VAS for the treatment of fetal lower urinary tract obstruction (LUTO) showed increased survival in babies undergoing fetal treatments but failed to identify any long-term benefits on the postnatal renal function [20].

The success of the fetal intervention highly depends on the proper selection of suitable candidates, which is hindered by the lack of reliable biomarkers of disease severity and progression [21].

Over the past few decades, many studies have investigated the use of demographic features, ultrasound findings, and fetal urinary analytes to prospectively predict the postnatal renal function and identify those fetuses that may benefit most from fetal intervention [18,22,23]. To date, however, the prognostic performance of these ultrasonographic parameters has shown contradictory results [22] and there is insufficient scientific evidence to recommend fetal analytes as biomarkers of kidney damage [23].

At birth, every baby with suspected PUV requires immediate bladder drainage to bypass the bladder obstruction.

A bladder and renal ultrasound scan should then be performed to confirm the antenatal findings and provide a baseline assessment with particular attention to renal development (renal dysplasia is a common finding particularly in the most severe cases).

The urinary drainage should be maintained until the neonate is stable enough to undergo the fluoroscopy test (micturating cystourethrogram: MCUG), that will confirm the diagnosis, and the endoscopic evaluation and, eventually, valve ablation [16].

Small paediatric cystoscopes and resectoscopes are available either to incise, ablate or resect the PUV, depending on surgeon's preference. However, extensive electrocoagulation should be avoided to prevent the formation of urethral strictures [16]. In case baby is too small or too unwell and depending on instrument availability, the resection of the valves can be postponed and a prolonged urinary diversion, obtained by maintaining the indwelling catheter or by performing a vesicostomy, could be considered until situation becomes more stable and baby is fit for the procedure.

The effectiveness of the initial valve ablation is confirmed by repeating a bladder and renal ultrasound scan and by fluoroscopic or endoscopic vision, depending on patient's clinical evolution and center's preference [16]. A decrease in the serum creatinine levels is also expected with the lowest value reached within the first year from valve ablation (nadir creatinine) considered a predictive value of long-term renal function [24].

However, in some of the most compromised patients, this initial management may not provide to be sufficient to relieve the high bladder pressure and alleviate the lower urinary tract symptoms.

For this reason, additional surgical procedures can be required.

The use of urinary diversion strategies for the management of PUV is one of the options, however, it still represents a controversial topic (**Figure 9.4**).

According to Krahn et al [25], cutaneous vesicostomy is an effective technique to protect the upper urinary tract, reduce the degree of the associated VUR and allow ureteral dilation to normalise.

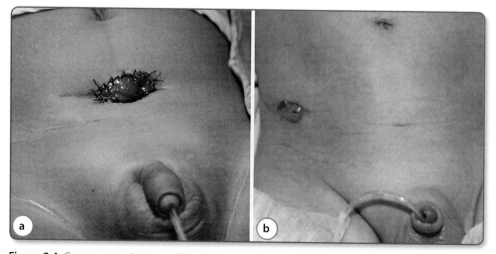

**Figure 9.4** Cutaneous vesicostomy (a) and right-side loop ureterostomy (b) in two male infants born with posterior urethral valves (PUV) (Evelina London Children's Hospital).

One of the controversies relates to the possibility that a urinary diversion can interfere with bladder compliance or capacity; Kim et al [26] and Sharifiaghdas et al [27] have reported that vesicostomy can be considered as a safe second-line treatment in case of compromised bladder, with little risk of further damaging.

Not only bladder procedures but also high urinary tract diversions have been considered valid surgical options to efficiently drain the upper urinary tract in children with PUV with poorly compliant bladders. The type of urinary diversion highly depends on surgeon's preference: high-loop ureterostomy, ring ureterostomy, and end-ureterostomy or pyelostomy have all been described, each showing advantages and disadvantages [16].

Neonatal circumcision should also be discussed with parents since the removal of the foreskin has proved to significantly decrease the incidence of UTIs in boys with PUV [28].

Antibiotic prophylaxis is also considered in order to prevent recurrent UTIs and protect the residual renal function, especially when a concomitant high-grade VUR is present [16].

## EARLY AND LONG-TERM MANAGEMENT

Life-long monitoring is mandatory for boys born with PUV to prevent long-term bladder and renal function deterioration.

Early valve ablation, in fact, does not always guarantee the preservation/restoration of a normal bladder and renal function. The pressures associated with the presence of an obstruction during the antenatal life can, in fact, significantly interfere with a normal bladder and renal development.

To assess the function of the upper urinary tract, serum creatinine levels, glomerular filtration rate, blood urea, nitrogen, and electrolytes should be periodically measured. Static renal scintigraphy with Tc-99m dimercaptosuccinic acid (DMSA) and dynamic renal scintigraphy with Tc-99m mercaptoacetyltriglycine (MAG3) are performed to monitor the split renal function and upper tract drainage.

The term 'valve bladder syndrome' has been introduced to define the pathophysiological changes occurring in the bladder of boys born with PUV after valve ablation.

It has been reported that PUV bladders undergo an initial phase of hypertrophy associated with an increase in the detrusor pressure and in a depressed urinary flow. The high bladder storage pressures are then transmitted back to the upper urinary tract with consequent renal tubular damage and nephrogenic polyuria. In a feedback loop, these high urinary volumes further impact an effective bladder dynamic, additionally increasing the post-void urine residual, and significantly affecting the function of the congenitally dysplastic kidneys.

Since this aspect is potentially modifiable, a close urological and nephrological follow-up is mandatory to prevent or delay bladder decompensation and renal deterioration.

Establishing correct voiding habits and introducing both behavioural and medical treatments together with a careful monitoring of the bladder function (urinary continence, bladder capacity, and post-void residual) have, therefore, a very important role.

Video-urodynamic studies are required to accurately assess bladder pressures and voiding dynamics; bladder overactivity and loss of bladder compliance could be present since the initial stages while myogenic failure associated with elevated post-void residual urine volumes are, usually, late findings [29].

Regarding behavioural management options, timed and frequent voiding, as well as double voiding, are recommended in selected cases to minimise the occurrence of bladder dysfunctions and UTIs.

In patients unable to completely empty their bladders, clean intermittent catheterisation (CIC) can be introduced to reduce post-voiding residuals. These can be performed through the native urethra or, in older children, through a Mitrofanoff appendicovesicostomy, which is often offered to those that are not compliant/cannot tolerate the passage of a catheter through their sensate urethra [30].

In addition, the use of an overnight catheter drainage is often indicated for preventing nocturnal bladder overdistension or urinary leaks, particularly for patients with polyuria or a very small bladder [16].

Apart from daytime CIC and overnight catheter drainage, the management of small capacity, overactive and/or high pressure bladders may also include anticholinergic drugs, that are also suggested to help preventing the remodelling of the bladder wall in the hypertrophy phase and delaying the occurrence of myogenic failure[29].

The use of alpha-adrenergic blockade drugs has been described to relieve secondary sphincteric hypertonicity, studies are currently investigating their role in the management of bladder neck obstruction in boys with PUV.

Other more invasive strategies, such as bladder neck incision, have also been described to improve bladder emptying, but their clinical utilities are still debated [31,32].

Finally, children with poorly compliant bladders with low capacity and high-filling pressures may ultimately require augmentation cystoplasty to preserve their upper urinary tract [29].

## OUTCOMES

Over the past few decades, the survival of boys born with PUV has significantly increased thanks to a better awareness of the pathology and its multi-systemic organ involvement, the spread of antenatal diagnosis and a multi-disciplinary approach.

While, in 1971, Johnston and Kulatilake [33] reported a mortality rate of 50.0%, in 1996, Dinneen and Duffy [34] described a dramatic improvement in the survival outcomes with a mortality rate of only 0–2%.

Improvements in prenatal diagnosis with early referrals to tertiary care paediatric hospitals, progress in perinatal management and in intensive care, and a better understanding of the aetiopathogenesis of bladder decompensation and renal function deterioration have surely contributed to improving the overall prognosis.

Long-term outcomes have been scarcely reported in children with PUV and only a few articles are currently available [35–38]. They suggest that lower urinary tract symptoms (LUTS) are two-times more frequently in young and middle-aged men with a previous history of PUV compared to the general population. In particular, urge and stress incontinence, hesitancy, weak stream, incomplete emptying, and straining are the most frequently reported complaining symptoms [34–38].

Particular attention has been given to long-term sexual function with encouraging reports that suggest good erectile function and normal fertility in adulthood, despite these men having various risk factors for sexual dysfunction including end-stage renal disease (ESRD), abnormal prostatic urethra, history of cryptorchidism, and recurrent epididymo-orchitis [36,37].

The outcome of renal transplant for PUV children developing ESRF is similar to other underlying conditions, in either long-term graft survival or renal function, providing adequate control of bladder function [36].

# CONCLUSION

Despite big progresses have been made in the understanding of the pathophysiology and the management of boys with PUV, a large proportion still experiences bladder and/or renal dysfunction.

A life-long follow-up by a multi-disciplinary team is, therefore, paramount for a proper management of children born with PUV to prevent bladder function deterioration and progression towards ESRF.

# REFERENCES

1. Bingham G, Rentea RM. Posterior Urethral Valve. StatPearls [Internet] 2021.
2. Brownlee E, Wragg R, Robb A, et al. Current epidemiology and antenatal presentation of posterior urethral valves: Outcome of BAPS CASS National Audit. J Pediatr Surg 2019; 54:318–321.
3. Capone V, Persico N, Berrettini A, et al. Definition, diagnosis and management of fetal lower urinary tract obstruction: consensus of the ERKNet CAKUT-Obstructive Uropathy Work Group. Nat Rev Urol 2022; 19:295–303.
4. Woolf AS, Thiruchelvam N. Congenital Obstructive Uropathy: Its Origin and Contribution to End-Stage Renal Disease in Children. Ad Ren Replace Ther 2001; 8:157–163.
5. Heikkilä J, Holmberg C, Kyllönen L, et al. Long-Term Risk of End Stage Renal Disease in Patients With Posterior Urethral Valves. J Urol 2011; 186;2392–2396.
6. Young HH, Frontz WA, Baldwin JG. Congenital Obstruction of the Posterior Urethra. J Urol 1919; 3:289–366.
7. Dewan PA, Keenan RJ, Morris LL, Quesne GWL. Congenital urethral obstruction: Cobb's collar or prolapsed congenital obstructive posterior urethral membrane (COPUM). Br J Urol 1994; 73:91–95.
8. Krishnan A, de Souza A, Konijeti R, Baskin LS. The Anatomy and Embryology of Posterior Urethral Valves. J Urol 2006; 175:1214–1220.
9. Tolmatschew N. Ein Fall von Semilunaren Klappen der Harn-rohre, und von Vergrosserter Vesicula Prostatice. Achiv Path Anat 1870; 348.
10. Bazy P. A propos du diagnostic de lesions renales unilaterales. Bull Mem Soc Chir Paris 1903; 101.
11. Wilckens KR. Zur Frage der Kongenitalen Stenosen der Mannlichen Harnrohre. Zeitschr F Urol 1910; 814.
12. Lowsley OS. Congenital malformation of the posterior urethra. Ann Surg 1914; 733.
13. Schreuder MF, van der Horst HJ, Bökenkamp A, Beckers GM, van Wijk JA Posterior urethral valves in three siblings: A case report and review of the literature. Birt Defects Res A Clin Mol Teratol 2008; 82:232–235.
14. Garriboli M, Ibrahim S, Clothier J. Spontaneous bladder rupture secondary to posterior urethral valves in a boy with Down syndrome. BMJ Case Rep 2021; 14:e240857.
15. Hodges SJ, Patel B, McLorie G, Atala A. Posterior Urethral Valves. Sci World J 2009; 9:1119–1126.
16. European Association of Urology. European Society for Paediatric Urology. EAU Guidelines; 2022. Available from https://uroweb.org/guidelines/paediatric-urology. (Last accessed 19th January 2023).
17. Morris RK, Middleton LJ, Malin GL, et al. Outcome in fetal lower urinary tract obstruction: a prospective registry study. Ultrasound Obstet Gynecol 2015; 46:424–431.
18. Lee J, Kimber C, Shekleton P, Cheng W. Prognostic factors of severe fetal megacystis. ANZ J Surg 2011; 81:552–555.
19. Ruano R. Fetal surgery for severe lower urinary tract obstruction. Prenat Diagn 2011; 31:667–674.
20. Morris RK, Malin GL, Quinlan-Jones E, et al. Percutaneous vesicoamniotic shunting versus conservative management for fetal lower urinary tract obstruction (PLUTO): a randomised trial. The Lancet 2013; 382:1496–1506.
21. Ruano R, Sananes N, Wilson C, et al. Fetal lower urinary tract obstruction: proposal for standardized multidisciplinary prenatal management based on disease severity: Prenatal classification of fetal LUTO. Ultrasound Obstet Gynecol 2016; 48:476–482.

22. Morris RK, Malin GL, Khan KS, Kilby MD. Antenatal ultrasound to predict postnatal renal function in congenital lower urinary tract obstruction: systematic review of test accuracy. BJOG Int J Obstet Gynaecol. 2009; 116:1290–1299.

23. Morris RK, Quinlan-Jones E, Kilby MD, Khan KS. Systematic review of accuracy of fetal urine analysis to predict poor postnatal renal function in cases of congenital urinary tract obstruction. Prenat Diagn. 2007;27:900–911.

24. Wu CQ, Blum ES, Patil D, Shin HS, Smith EA. Predicting childhood chronic kidney disease severity in infants with posterior urethral valve: a critical analysis of creatinine values in the first year of life. Pediatr Nephrol 2022; 37:1339–1345.

25. Krahn CG, Johnson HW. Cutaneous vesicostomy in the young child: indications and results. Urology 1993; 41:558–563.

26. Kim YH, Horowitz M, Combs A, et al. Comparative urodynamic findings after primary valve ablation, vesicostomy or proximal diversion. J Urol 1996; 156:673–676.

27. Sharifiaghdas F, Mirzaei M, Nikravesh N. Can transient resting of the bladder with vesicostomy reduce the need for a major surgery in some patients? J Pediatr Urol 2019; 15:379.e1–e379.e8.

28. Harper L, Blanc T, Peycelon M, et al. Circumcision and Risk of Febrile Urinary Tract Infection in Boys with Posterior Urethral Valves: Result of the CIRCUP Randomized Trial. Eur Urol 2022; 81:64–72.

29. Chan EP, Wang PZT, Dave S. Valve Bladder Syndrome Associated with Posterior Urethral Valves: Natural History, Work-up, and Management. Curr Bladder Dysfunct Rep 2020; 15:76–82.

30. King T, Coleman R & Parashar K Mitrofanoff for Valve Bladder Syndrome: Effect on Urinary Tract and Renal Function. J. Urol. 2014; 191, 1517–1522.

31. Singh SK, Sharma V, Singh A. Urodynamic Changes after Valve Fulguration Alone and Valve Fulguration with Bladder Neck Incision. J Indian Assoc Pediatr Surg 2019; 24:31–35.

32. Abdelhalim A, Hashem A, Abouelenein EE, et al. Can Concomitant Bladder Neck Incision and Primary Valve Ablation Reduce Early Re-admission Rate and Secondary Intervention? Int Braz J Urol 2022; 48:485–492.

33. Johnston JH, Kulatilake AE. The sequelae of posterior urethral valves. Br J Urol 1971; 43:743–748.

34. Dinneen MD, Duffy PG. Posterior urethral valves. Br J Urol 1996; 78:275–281.

35. Jalkanen J, Heikkilä J, Taskinen S. No single reason behind adult lower urinary tract symptoms in patients with posterior urethral valves. Scand J Urol 2019; 53:166–170.

36. Lopez Pereira P, Martinez Urrutia MJ, Espinosa L, Jaureguizar E. Long-term consequences of posterior urethral valves. J Pediatr Urol 2013; 9:590–596.

37. Taskinen S, Heikkilä J, Rintala R. Effects of posterior urethral valves on long-term bladder and sexual function. Nat Rev Urol 2012; 9:699–706.

38. Tikkinen KAO, Heikkilä J, Rintala RJ, Tammela TLJ, Taskinen S. Lower Urinary Tract Symptoms in Adults Treated for Posterior Urethral Valves in Childhood: Matched Cohort Study. J Urol 2011; 186:660–666.

# Chapter 10

# Paediatric speciality networks – a hub and spoke model of care

*Shelley Riphagen*

## INTRODUCTION

While the majority of children across the world are managed holistically by local paediatricians, there are occasions when specialist input and care are required. The fundamental question for specialised care is how to best deliver this type of care making specialised services readily available to the patient wherever they present, readily accessible to the referrer and in a manner which optimises outcomes, while improving clinical and economic efficiency. The foundation of the solution may lie in the anatomy of the referral network. Neonatal and adult critical care networks were established long before paediatrics followed. What have we learned in the United Kingdom (UK) along the way, and can the lessons be implemented globally?

## Background

Children between birth and 18 years make up <25% of the population of a country in the majority of developed nations including the UK [1]. The incidence of complex and critical illness in children varies from 13 to 27% depending on definitions [2] but is responsible for up to 10% of hospital admissions. It accounts for significant and disproportionate healthcare resource utilisation and up to around 40% of paediatric healthcare spend [3]. Critical illness in children in the developed world is a rare event with mortality rates having fallen over the past 30 years to between 2 and 3% [4]. Children with significant congenital structural and genetic defects, who would previously have died in early childhood are now surviving into later childhood and beyond with the help of access to innovative and improved treatments and services, including the use of respiratory support in the home setting. Along with increased survival of children with previously fatal conditions in early childhood, and the ability and facility to deliver home ventilation, parent, family and societal expectations have changed. The ability to provide long-term ventilatory support in the home for some conditions has resulted in the rapid increase in the number of children

**Shelley Riphagen** MB ChB Dip Obs (SA) FCP (paeds) SA, Evelina London Children's Hospital, Paediatric Intensive Care Consultant and Clinical Lead, South Thames Retrieval Service, Westminster Bridge Road, London, UK
Email: shelley.riphagen@gstt.nhs.uk

who are supported in this manner [5]. The consequence of caring for this burgeoning group of children with increasing complexity, and the necessity to ensure care for all sick children is delivered in the optimal location with the best outcomes, has increased the need to develop paediatric specialist networks across the world.

# BIRTH OF THE SPECIALIST PAEDIATRIC NETWORK IN THE UK

Up until the mid-1990s in the UK, very-low-frequency paediatric intensive care was undertaken occasionally by adult intensive care clinicians in district general hospital (DGH) settings. Paediatric anaesthesia and critical care had developed as a sub-speciality in the United States in the early 1990s [6]. Centralisation of paediatric intensive care provision quickly followed in many high-income countries. The impetus to centralise paediatric intensive care in the UK was propelled by evidence that the mortality for children in the UK, cared for in small numbers in adult intensive care units (AICU), was significantly higher than those with similar disease in Australia [7], and that higher volume centres (for many diseases) had improved outcomes in general. This led to the centralisation of paediatric intensive care units (PICU) and specialised paediatric services into the major cities in the UK. The result of this reduction in paediatric critical care providers from well over 1,000 DGH AICUs in the 1980s to under 30 PICUs by 2004, and the subsequent consolidation of care with the ability to ensure care was delivered by paediatric intensivists, resulted in an almost immediate improvement in mortality and subsequent annual ongoing improvement to align with the rest of the developed world within a short period of time, as seen in the PICANET annual report archive [8].

The centralisation of paediatric intensive care immediately created new challenges. Children presenting critically ill to their district general hospital needed to be resuscitated and stabilised by multi-disciplinary DGH teams which now had decreasing exposure to and experience with this group of children. Once resuscitated, children had to be transferred in optimal condition to the final destination PICU, anywhere from <10 to over 150 miles distant. There was clear evidence that teams' expert in transport medicine performed better than occasional operators with better outcomes and fewer critical incidents [9]. Arising from this need, the paediatric critical care transport teams were established in the UK. Over the past 20 years and following the same logic that increased volume improves outcome, the number of PCC transport teams in the UK has reduced from over 20 to 12 in 2022. Consolidation of some lower volume PCC transport services to combined PCC retrieval teams (PCCRT) has resulted in larger regions of care for the PCCRT than the PICU, and created the need to agree some management principles and commonalities, for example, for drug calculations and infusions. It was also necessary to develop PCC advice and support networks to enhance care delivered by local teams and ensure that critically ill children benefitted from high quality networked care delivered locally prior to and during attendance of the PCCRT [10,11]. The South Thames Retrieval Service (STRS) based in South London was the earliest adopter of this consolidated model and networked care in PCC in the UK. Established in 1997, it serves three paediatric intensive care units and a tertiary oncology service in South London transferring nearly 1,000 critically ill children per annum from 20 district general hospitals across the region. Soon after the establishment of STRS, it became clear that DGH-based teams needed more than just access to a paediatric emergency transfer service.

## EMERGENCY ADVICE AND CLINICAL SUPPORT

To optimise patient outcomes in the 'Golden hour' of resuscitation, the DGH teams needed access to emergency advice and clinical support to escalate to intensive care. In order to maintain essential skills and expertise and enhance team performance for these rare events for individual clinicians, there was also a need to develop education programmes and support of multi-disciplinary learning for recognition, stabilisation and resuscitation of the critically ill child. To facilitate optimal team working it was also necessary to have a specialist consultant 'friend' to phone – a clinical leader in the paediatric transport service who could act as a link for outreach education, audit feedback and service performance and review. Although the paediatric critical care services and transport teams had been centralised at the hub, it was necessary to develop outward reaching solid links to the DGH referrers to optimise performance at all levels including that of the retrieval service, to ensure it met the needs of the end-users – patients and referral teams. This practice ensures that patients, whilst still at smaller hospitals, have access to expert advice and can receive appropriate treatment directed by specialists with the potential to escalate as required. For the local paediatrician managing the child, there is an added layer of reassurance in the second opinion and specialist support. This not only helps in decision-making in the resuscitation and stabilisation of critically ill children, but also reduces clinical stress in local teams and may be beneficial from a legal stand-point as well. The attending paediatrician can concentrate on managing the child locally while the optimal destination centre, appropriate level of care and the safe transport of the child is secured by the PCC retrieval service.

Alongside the paediatric critical care developments, sub-speciality paediatric networks (for example, cardiology, neurosurgery, oncology and trauma among others) also developed, with referral patterns varying dependent on geography, institutional and personal loyalties and sub-speciality provision at the centralised tertiary paediatric centres. Although the paediatric sub-speciality clinical networks improved access to and quality of specialist care for children, the variation in referral patterns across specialties produced a confusing spider web of tertiary paediatric referral for many institutions, both at the referrer and receiver level. In an attempt to harmonise this, the National Health Service Commissioning Board published its strategy to develop operational delivery networks (ODN) in 2012 [12]. This document described how strategic clinical networks would be established to develop long-term strategy and improve outcomes, while ODNs would focus attention on standardising, simplifying, co-ordinating and improving access to care pathways. Although this added two organisational layers to the hub, the principle of hub and spoke care was maintained with an opportunity to harmonise referral patterns to reduce overlap and confusion, and potentially improve efficiency of access to the right care at the right time and place for every child (**Figure 10.1**).

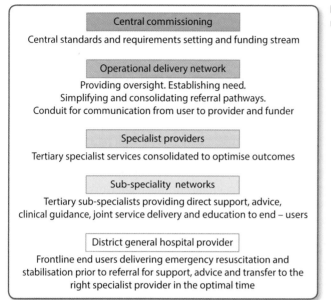

**Figure 10.1** Hub and spoke model of networks.

# DRIVING FORCE SUPPORTING NETWORKING

In 2018, the World Health Organization published an aspirational standard document to improve the quality of care delivered to children and adolescents around the world [13]. Experts from 88 countries agreed that among other important standards: all children should be receiving evidence-based medicine; children's healthcare data and informatics should be collected to evaluate and improve outcomes and that every child who presented with a condition that could not be managed optimally, at the site of presentation with the local available resources, should receive timely referral and safe transfer to a paediatric centre with enhanced expertise, to allow seamless continuity of care. The WHO endorsed the development of paediatric specialist referral networks for all countries, many of which already had established patterns of referral, but some without the organisational structure to optimise performance and minimise variation.

'Networking' by definition, as an arrangement of intersecting referral pathways, and 'group or system of inter-connected people or things' allows relevant information exchange and the development of professional contacts. These support improved access to the right care at the right time for children. In the UK and around the world, paediatric specialist networks and Paediatric ODNs are instrumental tools in the delivery of the WHO standards described above. In a strategy document 'Developing Operational Delivery Networks'. The way forward, in 2012, the NHS set out clearly the aims and goals of ODNs.

ODNs were to take a whole system overview of the region to ensure most clinically appropriate and sensible referral pathways for optimal clinical efficiency were established. These would ensure effective clinical flows through multi-professional provider collaboration and communication. Another goal was to improve consistency, reduce variation and improve service standards across the region in a manner that engaged all stakeholders. Additionally, a key role would be to review the geographic spread of resources, and support capacity planning with regard to staffed beds to accommodate the variations in activity imposed by seasonality in an attempt to match demand with capacity.

Paediatric ODNs focus on the bigger operational aspects of harmonising sub-speciality referral patterns within a region with the aim of improving quality and equity of care for children. Variations to access to the right care for children must be reduced, and care must be delivered at the right place and time for the acuity and nature of the condition with which the child presents. The ODN will try to ensure that standards are maintained and care is evidence-based across the region for all paediatric providers. This means facilitating development of shared sub-speciality evidence-based clinical guidelines, led by the experts; and supporting development of open lines of communication for seamless care. The remit is to support improvement in outcomes and quality standards for children based on agreed networked patient-care pathways.

The economic benefits of standardisation and improved efficiency are extremely important though without good data capture, difficult to evaluate.

Paediatric Specialist Networks as sub-groups working within the ODN provide sub-speciality support for DGH clinicians dealing with children with specific conditions. They develop condition specific guidelines for management of conditions which a DGH clinician may encounter only rarely, and they provide triage and advice after referral, for specialist consultation at the right time and place. The sub-speciality networks ensure that current evidence-based medicine can be applied to all children being referred, and that sub-speciality opinion and in some instances also delivery of care, from other regions and other parts of the world can be accessed in highly complex cases by all children who are referred. Sub-speciality consultants at the 'hub' tertiary centre are linked to each major referrer, providing a direct access conduit for professional advice and support, performance review, audit and two-way feedback. A child with epilepsy presenting to their local hospital can be managed by their local paediatrician with an interest in 'epilepsy' but also have access to specialist paediatric neurology for the management of a more complex presentation.

## TRAIL-BLAZERS: PAEDIATRIC SPECIALISED AND OPERATIONAL DELIVERY NETWORKS

The South Thames Paediatric Network (STPN) and the Yorkshire and Humber Paediatric Critical Care Operational Delivery network (Y&H PCCODN) were the first two paediatric ODNs in the UK to be established and supported by NHS specialised commissioning in 2018 as pilot projects. Their remit was to develop governance and reporting structures, establish funding needs and set out the strategy for the ODN going forward.

As trail blazers in this field, there was a need to engage stakeholders widely, understand in depth the complexity and challenges of paediatric care and referral, and establish the baseline of clinical care delivery at all levels of acuity.

Paediatric services in Greater London and the South East are historically extremely complex. STPN works collaboratively with 20 district general hospitals delivering acute paediatric care in hospitals across the South East of England, and four tertiary paediatric providers in London. These include the STPN-hosting or 'lead' centre at Evelina London Children's Hospital, Kings College Hospital and St George's Hospital with the Royal Marsden Hospital in Sutton providing tertiary paediatric oncology care, excluding critical care. Sub-speciality referral patterns are historically complex partly due to the delivery of tertiary paediatric care in London with seven out of eight providers within a 10-mile radius and none providing all aspects of tertiary paediatric care. The STPN has the ongoing task of trying to simplify referral pathways and ensure referral harmony between the paediatric sub-speciality networks with the ongoing need to review historic referral patterns and amend them in line with the majority where possible.

Prior to the establishment of the ODN, all major trusts operated independently with minimal commonality. Long-term ventilation (LTV), for example, was delivered using numerous devices across the region with no ability to bulk purchase or bulk train personnel. The development of the ODN and a specific group reviewing LTV across the region, for example, will allow improvement in standardisation and equity of training and support for this rapidly growing area of paediatrics.

The Y&H PCC ODN is almost equivalent in size and scope to STPN with 19 district general hospital sites and two tertiary paediatric providers. Their role is to co-ordinate patient pathways and ensure equitable access to specialist advice, support and resources. The ODN members work together to share expertise and learning is shared widely.

The development of various types of networks, of themselves a clinical management system, has necessitated a clear governance and reporting structure.

The P-ODN is hosted by a lead provider covering a defined region. The network is funded by and responsible to NHS Specialist commissioning with the remit to report activity, engage with contracting of services, monitor quality of service delivery, identify and escalate risks and support innovation.

The ODN is led and managed by experienced individuals who are part of a team employed by the host organisation for the purpose of delivering the P-ODN successfully. Within the ODN, paediatric sub-speciality networks deliver the care that the ODN facilitates, monitors and evaluates.

The ODN Board is comprised of a diverse group of individuals representing all aspects of the pathways of care for children from within the community to tertiary providers, commissioners and strategic network representatives and parents.

The ODN, responsible to NHS specialised commissioning, is required to report activity, expenditure and progress of goals. Although working together with stakeholders and providers to deliver improved care through standardisation, improved communication and service efficiencies, evaluating success is dependent on stakeholder engagement and evaluation of data.

Data submission and engagement is entirely stakeholder dependent with the ODN having no authority to enforce data submission or any of the clinical pathway changes suggested. The quality and consistency of data submission remains one of the biggest challenges.

There are myriad challenges facing the successful development and delivery of paediatric networks.

Developing a shared clinically relevant strategy that delivers improved care without apparently threatening providers is a major obstacle within the NHS, with whole-scale reform of services required to reduce duplication, simplify pathways and consolidate evidence-based care. The required change is disruptive and uncomfortable, and engaging in the discomfort of change voluntarily is rare.

Disentangling complex historic referral pathways from the emotional and institutional loyalties with which they are bound is painful to some, obscuring the long-term benefits of reform. It has frequently required multiple national service reviews to effect change in the UK. Children's cancer services and children's congenital heart services are just two of many more to mention.

Despite the fact that there is ample evidence that consolidated care of rare conditions improves outcomes, we as multi-disciplinary providers stand in the way of consolidation, because of the personal and institutional disruption it has to cause and despite the clinical and economic efficiencies and benefits it would bring. One of the roles of the ODN is to maintain institutional neutrality to ensure that the needs of the users (patients) are determined and an overview of the best delivery pathway of care maintained, with the goal to have this delivered in the simplest and most efficient manner, while ensuring harmony and co-operation between specialist care providers.

Data capture to evidence improvements in clinical care, efficiencies in service delivery or reduction in costs in a network is required in order for networks to be able to prove their benefit. There is no current uniform mechanism to capture this data across all specialties, with only paediatric critical care, cardiology and trauma having rigorous national data capture for audit. This ongoing deficiency in information technology resource and uniformity makes demonstrating value an ongoing challenge for network leaders.

## CONCLUSION

Networks have a major role as communication and collaboration conduits and can play a major role in bringing all stakeholders together to decide steps required to make incremental change towards the longer-term goal of meeting all the WHO standards for the care of sick children. The development of defined paediatric specialist referral networks established in a clinically and geographically sensible manner from the outset, facilitates the right care delivered at the right time while clinical teams present with the child, are fully supported by specialist advice delivered by experts who know and understand their working conditions, level of training and experience and the healthcare set up.

The development of paediatric specialist networks and more recently of the Paediatric ODNs in the UK has afforded the paediatric community, under the 'net' of the ODN, the means to work together as a wider team than in just departmental, speciality or institutional settings.

This bigger and better represented team has more power and combined means to effect bigger and more meaningful change for children and the wider NHS in a collaborative manner. To undertake this bigger task well, individuals involved and participating in the delivery of networks – at all levels – need time and space to develop mechanisms to effect strategic change in a manner that is the least personally and institutionally disruptive to its stakeholders but achieves the goal of delivering improved care for all children.

## REFERENCES

1.  Office for National Statistics. Population estimates for the United Kingdom, England and Wales, Scotland and Northern Ireland: Mid-2020. Census 2021.
2.  Wijlaars LPMM, Gilbert R, Hardelid P. Chronic conditions in children and young people: learning from administrative data. Arch Dis Childhood 2016; 101:881–885.
3.  Miller-Smith L, Finnsdóttir Wagner Á, Lantos JD. Epidemiology of Critical Illness in Children. Bioethics in the Pediatric ICU: Ethical Dilemmas Encountered in the Care of Critically Ill Children. International Library of Ethics, Law, and the New Medicine. Germany: Springer 2019;77.
4.  Demirkiran H, Kilic M, Tomak Y, et al. Evaluation of the incidence, characteristics, and outcomes of pediatric chronic critical illness. PLoS One 2021; 16:e0248883.
5.  McDougall CM, Adderley RJ, Wensley DF, Seear MD. Long-term ventilation in children: longitudinal trends and outcomes. Arch Dis Child 2013; 98:660–665.

6.  Epstein D, Brill J. A History of Pediatric Critical Care Medicine. Pediatr Res 2005; 58:987–996.

7.  Pearson G, Shann F, Barry P, et al. Should paediatric intensive care be centralised? Trent vs Victoria. The Lancet 1997; 349:1213–1217.

8.  PICANET annual report archive 2004 to 2020. Available from https://www.picanet.org.uk/annual-reporting-and-publications/annual-report-archive/ (Last accessed 21st January 2023).

9.  Ramnarayan P, Thiru K, Parslow RC, et al. Effect of specialist retrieval teams on outcomes in children admitted to paediatric intensive care units in England and Wales: a retrospective cohort study. The Lancet 2010; 376:698–704.

10. Seaton SE, Ramnarayan P, Davies P, et al. DEPICT Study Team. Does time taken by paediatric critical care transport teams to reach the bedside of critically ill children affect survival? A retrospective cohort study from England and Wales. BMC Pediatr 2020; 20:301.

11. Seaton SE, Draper ES, Pagel C, et al. The effect of care provided by paediatric critical care transport teams on mortality of children transported to paediatric intensive care units in England and Wales: a retrospective cohort study. BMC Pediatr 2021; 21:217.

12. NHS Commissioning Board. Developing operational delivery networks: the way forward 2012.

13. World Health Organization. Standards for improving the quality of care for children and young adolescents in health facilities. Available from https://www.who.int/publications/i/item/9789241565554. (Last accessed 21st January 2023).

# Chapter 11

# Safety checklists in paediatrics

*Marilyn McDougall*

## INTRODUCTION

Patient safety is a specific healthcare discipline necessary to prevent avoidable harm in an increasingly complex healthcare system. The Institute of Medicine published a report [1] entitled 'To Err Is Human: Building a Safer Healthcare System' in 2000 which shone the light on >95,000 patient deaths each year attributable to medical errors. The risk of death related to preventable errors is estimated to be 1 in 300 and up to 10% of patients suffer injury related to healthcare [2]. Patient safety incidents for children in hospital were associated with a '2–18-fold greater in-hospital mortality' according to a review by Miller et al in 2003 [3].

The nature of paediatric care has changed significantly due to advances in treatment and rising parental and societal expectations. Children are living dependant on technology including portable ventilators and high-risk medical treatment such as chimeric antigen receptor (CAR)-T therapy for cancer. But, these complex and high-risk therapies are inherently associated with more frequent and severe complications and require multiple teams working together to provide care. Healthcare providers are obliged to ensure that appropriate safety processes are in place to minimise the potential harm to patients.

One of the simplest and most cost-effective safety strategies which can be used in a wide variety of different setting is safety checklists. This chapter will explore the history of checklists, the evidence for their use in a variety of paediatric settings and the challenges associated with their implementation.

## HISTORY

Checklists are not unique to medicine. They are used to ensure that processes are completed in a standardised and systematic manner. Checklist can also improve team communication which is particularly important when individuals that do not routinely work together are required to perform urgent and time critical tasks.

One of the best-known safety checklists is the World Health Organisation (WHO) 'surgical safety checklist (SSC)' which was developed in 2008 to improve the safety of surgical care globally. The WHO SSC was developed by a group of experts including surgeons, anaesthetists, nurses, quality improvement experts and patients. Currently, >70% of

**Marilyn McDougall** MbChB FCPaed (SA) FRCPCH, Paediatric Intensive Care Unit, Evelina London Children's Hospital, London, UK
Email: marilyn.mcdougall@gstt.nhs.uk

operating rooms in 94 countries use the WHO SSC [4]. There are several reports and reviews demonstrating that use of the WHO SSC improves patient safety [4]. Most recently, a meta-analysis of implementation of the WHO SSC in low and middle-income countries by White et al [4] reported a 23% reduction in mortality and 44% reduction in complications. However, none of the reports were randomised controlled studies, in fact the majority ($n = 36$) were case reports.

THE WHO SSC has three components: 'sign in' before the induction of anaesthesia, 'time-out' before skin incision and 'sign out' before the patient leaves the operating theatre or procedure room. A checklist co-ordinator, usually the anaesthetist, ensures that all of the necessary teams including surgery, nursing and anaesthesia have completed the listed tasks before the operation can proceed. A key part of the checklist involves team members introducing themselves by name and stating their role, followed by the operator describing the operation and listing anticipated complications. By verbalising each of these stages, interdisciplinary communication is improved, the hierarchy is flattened and an opportunity is created for any team member, not just the leading surgeon, to question the procedure or plans.

Communication errors are responsible for a significant proportion of adverse events in healthcare. There is some evidence that non-technical skills (e.g. leadership, team working, communication, decision making, and situational awareness) are improved through utilisation of checklists. Checklists can also be used to improve the quality of information recorded in medical notes, administration of medication, and engagement of healthcare workers and families in patient care [3].

Checklists can incorporate mnemonics as an aide–mémoire to synthesise complex procedures and ensure that processes such as ward rounds are conducted in a comprehensive and systematic manner.

Although the WHO surgical safety checklist itself is simple, full team engagement and demonstration of the impact on patient safety are fundamental to sustained use of the checklist in any organisation. To date there is very little evidence regarding which implementation methods are most effective [4].

## SAFETY CHECKLISTS IN PAEDIATRIC SETTINGS

### Paediatric surgery

Incidences of congenital anomalies, trauma, cancers and acquired diseases continue to rise worldwide placing pressure on paediatric surgical services. The ability to perform complex operations on younger and smaller patient has led to improved childhood survival alongside higher risk and more complications. For decades, safe surgery focussed predominantly on intra-operative technique and decision-making [5]. The traditional hierarchy placed the surgeon as the leader with ultimate authority and responsibility. Despite the advances in surgical technique and equipment, too many patients have suffered unnecessary complications and suboptimal care. Research has demonstrated that safe and effective surgery requires evidence-based decision-making, multi-faceted treatment approaches to prevent complications, and effective communication in and out of the operating room.

In one study undertaken at a University Teaching Hospital in India [6], the checklist was used in 3,000 consecutive paediatric cases over a 2-year period. The checklists identified errors in describing the correct site of surgery in 108 cases (3.6%) which in 3 (0.15%)

cases could have led to major surgery on the wrong side. The investigators concluded that checklists provided a valuable prompt for the whole multi-disciplinary team involved to ensure all aspects of patient safety were appropriately addressed.

A study in a Nepal Medical College [7] found higher compliance with elective compared to emergency cases (49.7% vs. 13.4%) and no post-operative complications in fully compliant cases compared to 3.4% in partial or non-complaint cases reviewed. A total of 267 cases were included of which only 103 (38.6%) (35.6–41.6 at 95% confidence interval) were fully compliant with the checklist and a further 69 (25.8%) were partially compliant.

A process was designed for nationwide implementation of the WHO SSC in Benin [8]. The primary outcome was sustainability of checklist use at 12–18 months measured by a questionnaire. At 18 months, 86% of those surveyed reported compliance with the checklist compared to 31% before the training and 88% after 4 months. This was also associated with a significant improvement in patient safety culture as evidenced by increased Human Factors Attitude Questionnaire scores of 76.7, 81.1, and 82.2% before, and at 4 and 12–18 months after training respectively; ($p < 0.001$). Limitation of his study is that some of the results were based on self-evaluation using questionnaires and although there was also independent observation using the validated WHO BARS (WHO Behaviourally anchored rating scale), there was no control arm to the study.

A study conducted in the USA [9] demonstrated that despite good compliance with the WHO SSC up to 33% of specialist paediatric orthopaedic cases started without essential equipment in the operating theatre. This suggests that use of SSC alone does not prevent equipment failures in this setting, indicating that the WHO SSC may be insufficient to adequately prepare for some highly specialist operations.

## Ward rounds

Checklists can be used to improve family experience as well as patient safety. In a study conducted by Cox et al (2017) [10] the use of Family-Centred Rounds (FCR) Checklist was associated with improved family engagement and a more positive perception of the safety climate. This was a cluster-randomised trial involving 298 families. Two hospitals were randomised to use FCR checklists and two others delivered usual care. FCR intervention rounds were more likely to include asking family (OR = 2.43) or healthcare team (OR: 4.28) for questions.

## Emergency department

Intra-hospital transfers, particularly for children presenting to emergency departments (ED) requiring urgent admission to PCC are high risk episodes. 75% of reported ED adverse events or physiological deteriorations occur during these transfers [11]. In one hospital, a novel checklist was created using the mnemonic BETTER (Briefing ED-to-ICU Transport To Exit Ready) to improve the safety of these transfers [11]. The authors reported a high checklist completion rate (84%, 335 out of 400 PICU medical admissions) and 87% of nurses and 93% of physicians agreeing that the BETTER checklist improved patient safety during transfer. They were also able to demonstrate a 78% relative reduction in intra-hospital transfer (IHT) incidents in this area of the hospital, consistent with prior reports of 41–68% reduction of IHT incidents using checklists [11]. The limitations of this particular study were that it was confined to a single children's hospital in the United States and that the observers were not blinded to the intervention.

## Critical care

The paediatric critical care (PCC) setting is a particularly high-risk area. According to a literature search, the number of adverse events or complications per 100 days in PCC ranges from 2.7 to 33 [12]. The use of cognitive tools such as checklists can be effective in these settings.

At Children's Hospital of Eastern Ontario (CHEO) [13] 17-points checklist was devised which took <2 minutes to complete. A trained research assistant attended the PCC ward-rounds to assess compliance with the checklists from September 2013 to February 2014. They reported 89.2% compliance in 132/148 rounds observed (95% CI: 83.2–93.2%). Use of the checklist led to a change in patient care in 69/132 events [95% CI: 44.2–61%].

The 'KIDS SAFE checklist for Paediatric Intensive Care' [12] developed in Brisbane, Australia focusses on the methodology required to design a bespoke checklist suited to PCC. The authors emphasise the use of a short and memorable mnemonic to make it easier to recall the items on the checklist. The one they create is entitled KIDS SAFE and includes 'eight areas: kids developmental needs, infection, deep vein prophylaxis, skin integrity, sedation, analgesia, family, and enteral feeding'. This differs from FASTHUG that is used in many adults ITU through inclusion of developmental needs and family and exclusion of items such as glycaemic control which has less evidence than in adult care [12].

However, not all studies demonstrate a positive benefit form checklist implementation. One study undertaken in New York by Sahulee et al [14] was designed to detect a 10% reduction in non-essential central venous catheter (CVC) days. The study was conducted between June 2013 and December 2017 during which 778 CVC days were placed for a total of 7,947 days. Statistical process control charts were used to analyse the quarterly mean and post-operative CVC duration. Unfortunately rather unexpectedly, the study demonstrated an increase in mean CVC duration after implementation of the safety checklist.

## Medication – compliance and safety

A Cochrane review [15] of interventions to reduce medication errors included seven controlled studies, one of which focussed on the implementation of a checklist. Although all seven studies aimed to improve medication safety for children, not all interventions targetted specific paediatric safety issues. Many of the studies were undertaken in a large teaching hospital and may not be generalisable. The review also highlighted the lack of investigations and research focussing on medication safety strategies for children.

Lépée et al 2012 implemented a check and control checklist to identify technical and clinical errors in prescriptions in a London, UK teaching hospital [16]. The checklist highlighted specific features of paediatric pharmaceutical care, such as weight-based dosages or routes of administration. They were able to demonstrate an improvement in the quality of prescriptions without any significant change on patient outcomes. Structured prescribing forms might improve prescribing practices in general, as shown by Kozer 2005 [17]. In this small study, randomised study conducted over an 18-day period there were 2,157 visits to ED. Use of the structured from was associated with a reduction in risk OR: 0.55 (95% CI: 0.34–0.99) in the 376 (16.6%) of orders compared to the 411 (52.2%) using the standard prescriptions.

## Coronavirus disease 2019

During the coronavirus disease 2019 (COVID-19) pandemic, a group of experts from leading organisations in the USA met to review the SSC in the light of the COVID-19 pandemic [18]. The purpose of the meeting was to improve patient and healthcare provider safety in operating theatres during the pandemic. They demonstrated that although the SSC is a universally acceptable tool it can easily be adapted in particular situation.

The group were able to reach consensus regarding nine modifications to the checklist such as checking the patient's COVID test results, reviewing the aerosolisation risk of the procedures and ensuring that appropriate personal protective equipment was available for all theatre staff. They also reviewed the process necessary to implement the changes such as identifying local leadership for the programme and including COVID-specific team simulation training. The need for regular review and revision as the pandemic progressed and de-implementation was also carefully considered.

# CHALLENGES

Although checklists are cost-effective and simple tools with extensive evidence to support their benefit in a wide variety of settings, there are also many studies demonstrating that both compliance and utilisation wanes over time.

Studies in paediatric operating theatres, wards and critical care units show poor compliance [19,20]. A Canadian study was conducted to identify the reasons for lack of enthusiasm or compliance with surgical checklists. Reasons identified in this study included the 'top-down' mandated nature of surgical safety checklist, lack of perceived benefit and redundancies with other surgical processes as possible contributing factors.

In addition to compliance with checklists, utilisation quality of the application and fidelity with the process is essential. This was effectively demonstrated by Anderson et al [19] who conducted a study of intra-operative delays and correlated them with fidelity and purposeful adherence to the SSC. In this study, trained observers monitored SSC compliance during 2014–2016. A total of 591 cases were observed and 19% ($n = 110$) had at least one documented, intra-operative delay. The majority of delays were related to missing (50%) or malfunctioning (30%) equipment. Compared with cases without delays, cases with delays did not have a different mean degree of adherence ($96.3 \pm 7.6\%$ vs. $95.6 \pm 5.8\%$, $P = 0.36$). However, the degree of fidelity was different between cases with and without delays (mean fidelity $77.1 \pm 14.9\%$ vs. $80.5 \pm 14.3\%$, $P = 0.03$).

# FUTURE RECOMMENDATIONS

In order for checklists to achieve the goal of reducing morbidity and mortality in paediatric care it is necessary to maintain compliance and engagement. This can be achieved by 'buy in' at all levels from the most senior to junior members of staff. Including the relevant teams in design of the checklist has been shown to support their implementation [10,11,13], but it is also necessary for senior managers to address issues identified by checklists to sustain their utilisation.

Checklists need to be easy to conduct or remember, using simple mnemonics, so that they can be repeated without causing unnecessary delays in busy and stressful environments. They also need to be tailored to the patient population and specialised procedures to maximise their benefit. When appropriately implemented they can reduce unwarranted errors such as wrong site surgery and medicine administration errors. This chapter demonstrates their versatility with examples of utilisation in every continent and a wide range of settings from ED and ward to PCC and operating theatres. The ongoing promotion and appropriate modification of safety checklists for paediatric care is an important cost-effective patient safety that should continue to be promoted widely.

## CONCLUSION

- Advances in treatment have led to a steady improvement in survival of children in hospital. However these advances are associated with increased complexity of care , more incidents and rising costs of treatment. Safety checklists are a simple, cost effective way of reducing harmful incidents which are associated with 12–18 fold increased in-hospital mortality. Checklists can be used to improve multi-disciplinary team working, flatten hierarchy  and optimise team working in complex environments such as operating theatres. They can be implemented to improve quality of prescriptions and safety transferring children between different departments. They have also been used in paediatric ward and intensive care environments to improve ward-round communication with bedside nurse and parents.
- Relevant teams should be involved in the design of local checklists. Tailoring checklists to a specific environment and patient population can be quickly and effectively achieved as demonstrated by modification of the SSC for COVID-19.
- Without active participation and good adherence checklists alone do not improve patient safety. Issues identified by checklists need to be addressed to avoid ongoing harm. The benefits of checklists need to be regularly demonstrated to users and their implementation supported by organisational leaders to maximise their impact.

## REFERENCES

1. Institute of Medicine. To Err Is Human: Building a safer Healthcare system [Internet]. Washington, DC: National Academies Press, 2000. Available from https://www.nap.edu/catalog/9728/to-err-is-human-building-a-safer-health-system [Last accessed 18th January 2023].
2. The Lancet. Patient safety: too little, but not too late. The Lancet [Internet] 2019; 394:895.
3. Miller MR, Elixhauser A, Zhan C. patient safety events during pediatric hospitalizations. Pediatrics 2003; 111:1358–1366.
4. White MC, Randall K, Capo-Chichi NFE, et al. Implementation and evaluation of nationwide scale-up of the Surgical Safety Checklist. Br J Surg [Internet] 2019; 106:e91–e102.
5. Mahmood T, Mylopoulos M, Bagli D, Damignani R, Aminmohamed Haji F. A mixed methods study of challenges in the implementation and use of the surgical safety checklist. Surgery 2019; 165:832–837.
6. Oak S, Dave N, Garasia M, Parelkar S. Surgical checklist application and its impact on patient safety in pediatric surgery. J Postgraduate Med [Internet] 2015; 61:92.
7. Bajracharya J, Shrestha R, Karki D, Shrestha A. Compliance of WHO surgical safety checklist at a pediatric surgical unit in a tertiary level hospital: A descriptive cross-sectional study. J Nepal Med Assoc 2021; 59:1256–1261.
8. White MC, Peven K, Clancy O, et al. Implementation strategies and the uptake of the World Health Organisation surgical safety checklist in low and middle income countries: a systematic review and meta-analysis. Ann Surg 2021; 273:e196–e205.

9.  Thomasson BG, Fuller D, Mansour J, Marburger R, Pukenas E. Efficacy of surgical safety checklist: Assessing orthopaedic surgical implant readiness. Healthcare 2016; 4:307–311.
10. Cox ED, Jacobsohn GC, Rajamanickam VP, et al. A family-centered rounds checklist, family engagement, and patient safety: A randomized trial. Pediatrics [Internet] 2017; 139:e20161688.
11. Venn AM-R, Sotomayor CA, Godambe SA, et al. Implementation of an intrahospital transport checklist for emergency department admissions to intensive care. Pediatr Qual Saf 2021; 6:e426.
12. Ullman A, Long D, Horn D, Woolsley J, Coulthard M. The KIDS SAFE checklist for pediatric intensive care units. Am J Crit Care 2022; 22:61–69.
13. McKelvie B, McNally JD, Menon K, et al. A PICU patient safety checklist: rate of utilization and impact on patient care. Int J Qual Health Care. 2016; 23:371–375.
14. Sahulee R, Ramirez MM, Al-Qaqaa YM, Chakravarti SB, McKinstry J. Safety checklist implementation did not reduce central venous catheter duration in pediatric cardiac ICU patients. Pediatr Qual Saf 2020; 5:e253.
15. Maaskant JM, Vermeulen H, Apampa B, et al. Interventions for reducing medication errors in children in hospital. Cochrane Database Syst Rev [Internet] 2015: CD006208.
16. Lépée C, Klaber RE, Benn J, et al. The use of a consultant-led ward round checklist to improve paediatric prescribing: An interrupted time series study. Eur J Pediatr 2012; 171:1239–1245.
17. Kozer E. Using a preprinted order sheet to reduce prescription errors in a pediatric emergency department: A randomized, controlled trial. Pediatrics 2005; 116:1299–1302.
18. Panda N, Etheridge JC, Singh T, et al. We Asked the Experts: The WHO surgical safety checklist and the COVID-19 pandemic: recommendations for content and implementation adaptations. World J Surg 2021; 45:1293–1296.
19. Anderson KT, Bartz-Kurycki MA, Masada KM, et al. Decreasing intraoperative delays with meaningful use of the surgical safety checklist. Surgery. 2018 Feb;163(2):259-263.
20. Bartz-Kurycki MA, Anderson KT, Abraham JE, et al. Debriefing: the forgotten phase of the surgical safety checklist. J Surg Res 2017; 213:222–227.

# Chapter 12

# Shaping health futures in the new digital age

*Anil Krishnaih, Gautam Kulkarni*

## INTRODUCTION

Healthcare is experiencing a digital revolution. The proliferation of hand-held and wearable digital health technologies, tele-healthcare capabilities including the tech-enabled virtual wards are promoting remote monitoring, instant access to information and self-care abilities for individuals. These empowered patients are seeking health information by researching online, understand their conditions better and write and read reviews about their doctors or hospitals for making better informed choices about their health and well-being needs. These emerging forces in the healthcare market ecosystem are redefining how healthcare services are now sought and offered [1].

Rapid progress in computing capabilities with cloud technologies and the coronavirus disease (COVID) pandemic have helped to accelerate the creation of digital front door [2] in healthcare, offering patients a new connected experience in their healthcare journey. Conversational artificial intelligence (AI) is fast becoming one of the key pillars of this digital front door deployed as personalised virtual assistant, an intelligent bot as real-time symptom checker tool and to automate administrative processes and engage users in human-like conversations.

With most healthcare services are still offered in the physical environment of hospitals, a new mobile-first, 'Phy-gital' model, an extended reality technology is making entry in the healthcare industry, offering patients new experiences in which the physical and digital components converge driving the newer expectations and experiences. The healthcare industry is not immune to the 'Amazon Effect'; as a result, healthcare needs are becoming more complex. Transformative digital technology innovations in other industries (e-commerce, banking, and many other service industries) are disrupting the conventional physical retail locations, redefining consumer preferences and directly influencing the patients' expectations and the way healthcare service providers respond to their demands.

**Anil Krishnaih** MBBS MRCPCH DCH MSc (Health Economics and Policy) Clinical Informatician, Member of FCI (Faculty of Clinical Informatics) Former Clinical Lead at NHS Digital, Medical Director, Capri Healthcare, Paediatric Intensivist at Cromwell Hospital, London, UK
Email: anil.me@icloud.com

**Gautam Kulkarni** MD DNB FRCPCH Dip Allergy, Consultant in Paediatrics and Adolescent Health The Portland Hospital London, Circle Health and Nuffield Health; Health Tech Adviser, London, UK
Email: drgkulkarni@gmail.com

This represents a significant shift from the traditional 'derived demand' model, where the needs of a patient are determined by their healthcare professionals, to an 'on-demand model, where people seek instant access to services anytime from anywhere based on their perception of needs. While many of the health issues will continue to be challenging to manage, advances in genomics in routine healthcare will enhance disease prediction, risk stratification, diagnosis and treatment of illnesses and transform the current model of healthcare to be more proactive, upstream, and predictive [2–4].

Connected health, mobile technology, artificial intelligence (AI), and big data are making a significant difference in how patients are diagnosed, treated, and managed. However, the *sine qua non* of lasting digital transformation fundamentally lies in the cultural shift across all stakeholders within the healthcare ecosystem. Therefore, clinicians and healthcare leaders must understand and embrace modern technologies in healthcare and influence how these technologies are harnessed and rethink the innovative ways how services should be designed and delivered.

'The Topol Review – Preparing the healthcare workforce to deliver the digital future' has observed that 90% of all jobs in the National Health Service (NHS) in the next 20 years will require healthcare professionals to be digitally skilled enough to navigate a data-rich healthcare environment. To achieve this, the workforce would need to possess an appropriate level of digital literacy; an understanding of the ethical challenges with the broader adoption of genomics and other digital technologies; a capacity for innovation; and an ability to address problems in an agile and flexible way [5,6].

The review recommendations go further to say that the rapid rate of changes in healthcare knowledge has spawned challenges for regulators, clinicians, and educators to identify what are the future relevance skills for the young professionals and the areas currently taught that could be safely omitted from future programmes. With access to mobile learning and other advanced cognitive learning experiences (Extended reality tools like AR and VR), there is a need to define how and what information medical trainees and professionals need to know and what information they need to be aware of but not necessarily to memorise [5].

The field of 'clinical informatics, genomic sciences, artificial intelligence, digital medicine, robotics would be redefining clinicians' roles, responsibilities, and expectations over the next two decades. In this context, health organisations and academia need to equip themselves to bridge the knowledge gap between the current and the future workforce and align their programmes to drive digital competency skills.

Organisations such as EFMI (European Federation of Medical Informatics), AAMI (American Medical Informatics Association), FCI UK (Faculty of Clinical Informatics), and Mobilising Computable Bioinformatics Knowledge (MCBK) are all driven by the professional communities and provide education, training, accreditation, and certification for the next generation clinicians to become skilled informatics professionals. Recently, FCI UK has designed a 'Core Competency Framework' defining the principles, core knowledge and skills-based competencies for clinical informaticians and through which these competencies can be mapped to educational and professional initiatives [7,8].

# DECODING THE 'DIGITAL HEALTH' COSMOS

Digital Health is an interdisciplinary domain that blends healthcare with information technology to enhance healthcare delivery and outcomes. It constitutes all technological solutions that engage patients and the healthcare providers. Such solutions include m-health (mobile-health), electronic health records (EHR), telemedicine, clinical decision support systems (CDSS) using artificial intelligence (AI) and machine learning (ML) tools, wearables with embedded sensors technology, IoT, augmented and virtual reality, digital medicines, and digital therapeutics (DTx) [7].

*Digital medicine* refers to using technologies as tools for measurement and intervention in the health of individuals and is driven by high-quality hardware and software applications that support the practice of medicine. These products can be used independently or in concert with pharmaceuticals, biologics, devices, or other products to optimise patient care and health outcomes [8,9].

*Digital therapeutics* provide evidence-based, software-driven therapeutic interventions to prevent, manage or treat medical disorders or diseases. Some of these are clinically prescribed [10,11] as therapeutics. VR is used as DTx tool in the management of chronic pain.

*SaMD*: Software applications used for medical purposes and performing these purposes without being part of a hardware medical device are classified as Software as Medical Devices (SaMD) [12]. This software is not similar to the software that is integral to a medical 'Device' and is rather classified as 'Software' in a 'Medical' device. SaMDs perform various clinical functions across diagnosis, automated triaging, monitoring and therapeutic interventions, using data generated from wearables to EMR, etc. With such software, even a single issue with design, implementation, usage, or functionality would introduce significant clinical risks as a result of incorrect decisions, which impacts on patient safety.

Health IT applications including these technologies prior to going live, need rigor around clinical risk management at an early stage of development, undergo regulatory oversights and approvals with 'reasonable assurance for clinical safety and effectiveness' for the intended clinical purposes. Assurance principles aim to ensure all stakeholders, including regulators, promote safe innovation and protect patient safety [13].

The actual power of digital technologies in healthcare will be realised only when the multiple siloed systems that capture data within and across care organisations can exchange data in timely and in clinically meaningful way. Various clinical terminology (e.g. SNOMED CT), content (PRSB in UK), and transport standards (HL7, FHIR) are promoting standardised and effective exchanging of health information between systems.

Just as the internet's capability is enabled by common standards through which all browsers and email clients exchange information, connecting the heterogeneous health information systems and leveraging open standards to enable syntactic and semantic interoperability remains critical [14]. Such a level of true interoperability improves patient care and staff experiences, enabling better-integrated care by making the right information available at the right time and at the right place. This will improve patient safety through reduced clinical errors, empower people to access their information and support the use of data for research, population health and policymaking [15].

# DIGITAL HEALTH TECHNOLOGY IN PAEDIATRIC LANDSCAPE

From preventive care to point of care, the way the services are delivered in paediatrics is being disrupted by data-driven science and innovations in digital health technologies. A glimpse into a few of the innovative trending technologies only reveals the immense possibilities evolving around us.

- Nanotechnology is used for innovative targeted drug delivery methods, imaging techniques, in minitablets, Oro-dispersible films and in monitoring devices to manage extreme premature babies and childhood blood disorders, cystic fibrosis, etc. [16–19].
- Advanced data science applications in pharmacogenomics and bioinformatics have found new ground-breaking therapies that cure, delay, or prevent certain conditions like childhood cancers, Type 1 diabetes, muscular disorders, epilepsy, end-stage renal disease and IBD. Predicting adverse reactions to medications is now possible using genetic information, enabling clinicians to select individualised therapies based on disease conditions and individual patient profiles.
- Three-dimensional (3D) printing and bioprinting in paediatrics are revolutionising paediatric care, especially seen in surgical planning, prosthetics, tissue constructs, and drug printing. In addition, 3D printing of medicines offers dose individualisation for paediatric medicines with varying dosages, sizes, release profiles and drug combinations improving medication compliance and adherence [20].
- Virtual and augmented reality technology are used in the management of paediatric pain and anxiety during certain day-care procedures and also in gamification as part of behavioural management tools with teenagers.
- Healthcare robots in the form of clinical robots (e.g. help in surgery and diagnosis), assistive robots (e.g. patient lifting and aiding in routine services) and rehabilitation robots.
- Humanoid social robots are being explored to address the emotional aspects of hospitalised children. This technology has shown some promising results [21].
- Rehabilitation robots are designed to restore the functionality and mobility of those with physical disabilities. Advanced wearable technology is revolutionising paediatric rehabilitation. Virtual reality games using VR headsets are used in physiotherapy and occupational therapy sessions; 3D motion-analysis sensors and software for analysing gait and limb movement are deployed to develop splinting and orthopaedic surgery guidelines. In addition, augmented communication technologies, such as eye-tracking devices for operating digital communication platforms for children with neuromuscular disorders are becoming part of rehabilitation programme.
- Undoubtedly, data-driven care is transforming our understanding of diseases, disease burden, innovative diagnostics solutions, the effectiveness of therapeutic interventions, and standardisation of care. The application of AI as a clinical decision support tool is not just providing optimism in clinical care but also in research and development (R&D), pharmaceutical and other innovations to offer precision diagnostics, care, and interventions. For example, researchers at Cedars–Senai have developed an AI model that can predict with 87% accuracy how a woman would deliver within 4 hours of being admitted to the hospital. By embedding this model into an electronic medical record, the model could aid professionals caring for their patients in making better decisions and reduce uncertainty from the labour and birth experiences.
- A deep-learning algorithm that primarily uses surface area information from magnetic resonance imaging of the brain of 6–12-month-old individuals is able to predict the diagnosis of autism in individual high-risk children at 24 months (with a positive predictive value of 81% and a sensitivity of 88%) [21].

# FUTURE OF HEALTHCARE AND THE ROLE OF GOVERNMENT

The overarching aim of 'Digital Health' is to promote health and well-being for everyone, everywhere. The development of future technologies remains predictably unpredictable. In this context, digital health transformation is not limited to technology existing tools such as – smartphones, mobile apps, wearables, and web-based hospital systems alone.

The national digital information infrastructure for health developed over the last decade in many countries was intended at collecting, storing, and sharing data. These are now undergoing rapid modernisation and the gateway for nationwide health information network are being developed in many countries. With advances in data sciences and the development of open standards, the data generated in the ever more heterogenous Health IT systems are transformed and transmitted as structured data formats. Such structured data models enable the clinical information systems to interoperate in such a way that the data can be effectively retrieved, processed and meaningfully interpreted for the purposes of direct care and promote reporting and optimisation of the data-driven quality, safety, and efficiencies in healthcare services.

As technology rapidly evolves, there is an urgent need to overhaul the structures, policies and institutions that govern health systems. Health is increasingly becoming more quantified while we start to see considerable benefits from the datafication of health. However, poor governance and data standards pose significant risks to patients' lives [22–24]. This risk presents an immediate opportunity for policy experts to address data governance, cyber security related concerns and to develop agreed ethical frameworks.

A genuine digital transformation of the healthcare system is a political choice. Recently more countries including India, Brazil and other South Asian countries are joining Sweden and Denmark. Israel, the UK, and the UAE, the leading global exemplars of digital health strategy in designing their own national digital health strategies. There is a need to transform the operating models at a scale to generate rapid value from digital transformation to promote patient-centred, value-based care models at national and at organisation levels. The government's role is to legislate, implement national digital health policies, develop an overall health economy framework, and regulate the market to create an ecosystem where innovation can flourish for the safe, effective, and most useful ideas to be adopted and scaled at pace.

# INTERFACING PAEDIATRICIANS WITH CLINICAL INFORMATICS

Clinical informatics is a non-orthodox clinical specialty, currently offered as a certified programme with unique clinician training paths in many countries. In its simplest terms, clinical informatics is the application of information and technology knowledge for capturing the data in practice in a clinically meaningful way and apply this to drive operational efficiencies, patient experiences and outcomes. Knowing this field exists is important, and trainees can now explore this specialty early in their career. The healthcare industry remains conventionally risk-averse and suffers from hierarchical challenges. This would make an effective change management particularly more arduous. Clinicians have unique expertise and ingenuity in solving issues in healthcare and with their ability to analyse and mitigate patient risks. Clinical leadership and their knowledge about informatics are critical for the safe and effective deployment of the systems. The professional bodies should leverage their lobbying power to promote effective digital health adoptions by wider enterprises, patients, and fellow professionals.

Having a clinical voice built into the discovery, design and implementation of health IT systems ensures the products' usability, clinical safety and effectiveness. Data driven tools such as Clinical Decision Support Systems (CDSS) augment healthcare providers in a variety of decisions and patient care tasks through provision of alerts and reminders, evidence-based recommendations, image recognition, diagnostic assistance, and therapy planning all centered around the patients. [25]. Use of such tools can introduce unintended consequences from automation biases and inadvertently contributing to serious errors. Clinicians have opportunities now to train in the principles of safety, risk management and risk mitigation in the manufacture and implementation of health IT systems.

Technology should become an asset for clinical practice and not a barrier; technology should work for us and help in releasing more time for clinicians to care for their patients. As paediatricians, in our practices, we spend a great deal of time carrying out many consultations every day. Therefore, to be productive, a technology solution that works for a practice should be leveraged and streamline the clinical workflow and practice operations.

Healthcare is changing dramatically, health IT systems are going to play a larger role, and the need for clinicians to understand the basics of principles of clinical informatics and the importance of data-driven delivery of healthcare across the domains of services, products and outcomes are paramount. The new model of care is becoming data-centric with increasing reliability on data analysis for prediction and prevention. The field is wide open with many exciting tech projects on the horizon and underway making the healthcare future more exciting. The future is digital and has only just begun!

## HOW DO WE TRANSLATE A VISION INTO REALITY?

We focus as a case study on RESCAPE, a virtual reality device, in understanding how it was developed to help paediatric patients. Early work in the field was developed by Dr. Hoffman, who has been exploring ways to use immersive VR for pain control since 1996 [26]. One area of his work that has received particular attention is the use of VR to help reduce the pain and distress of burn injuries in children. Dr Hoffman has used VR to address this issue is by developing immersive virtual environments that can distract children from the pain they are experiencing [27].

In the UK, RESCAPE has developed an immersive therapeutic treatment solution called DR. VR which was designated the first VR class 1 medical device in the UK in December 2020. It is showing considerable benefits within paediatric care and is being used extensively by play care specialists to reduce anxiety before and during procedures [28].

RESCAPE has adopted the Design Council's double diamond design methodology [29] for creating a new product. The double diamond methodology defines four phases of a project (**Figure 12.1**).

- *Discover*: An open phase where the team is encouraged to explore an issue and bring fresh and deep insight to the problem.
- *Define*: The creative research within the 'discover phase' is defined and refined into a brief and set of questions that can be easily explained.

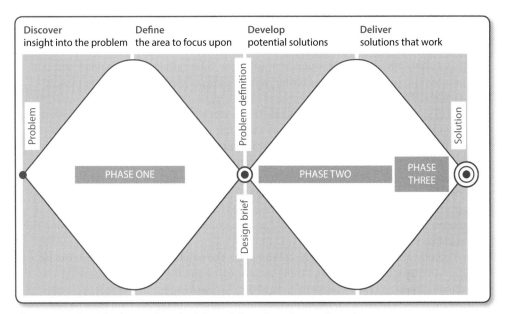

**Figure 12.1** Double-diamond methodology defines four phases of a project.

- *Develop*: With a defined brief the team can set about creating potential solutions that fulfil the brief.
- *Deliver*: Potential solutions are reviewed and combined to create a final solution that can be deployed and tested.

Working with clinicians, RESCAPE has developed three types of immersive content that can be tailored to the specific needs and preferences of different patients.

1. *Escape*: Highly immersive experiences using audio and 360 visuals to distract patients from their pain and anxiety. Patients can enjoy an African safari, get up close to dinosaurs or go to space and travel across the universe.
2. *Distract*: Highly immersive games that require the patient to direct the flow of the experience and avoid obstacles in order to score points.
3. *Relax*: A choice of relaxation spaces set in different serene environments. Users take part in guided breathing exercises featuring relaxing imagery and calming audio. This reduces anxiety in adolescent and paediatric patients using established breathing exercises.

For immersive therapies to fully live up to its potential, clinical teams must embrace the technology. As the technology that delivers 'Virtual Reality' is moving fast, consumer VR headsets like the 'Meta Quest' are becoming more advanced and widely available, and the content that is being created for these platforms is becoming more diverse and sophisticated.

The use of VR is now being explored in mental health, such as prolonging attention spans for ADHD [30]. As the technology continues to evolve, it is likely that we will see even more innovative and impactful uses of VR in the future with it being used not only in physical rehabilitation and becoming common place in use before, during and after procedures, but also in improving concentration in neuro-developmental conditions. This is a classic example of clinicians working with industry to deliver products best suited for our patients!

# CONCLUSION

- Healthcare is changing dramatically, and clinicians have a critical role in ensuring that digital health initiatives are grounded in evidence-based practice, are patient-centric, equitable and prioritise ethical considerations, data privacy, and security to protect patients' rights.
- OpenAI' ChatGPT in healthcare could take the world by storm, and the role of AI in healthcare is no longer a science fiction story. It is possible, patient consultations and even notes from EPR are interpreted and summarised by this AI tool, which prepares discharge summaries and automatically completes a referral. Furthermore, based on the summary of the consultation/discharge records, it searches for relevant patient information and guides patients to manage their health better. Recently ChatGPT performed at or near passing threshold on USMLE exams and may soon start writing chapters like this in journals, and could act as a mentor for healthcare researchers. The possibilities are endless from here on.
- As digital health and data continue to transform the paediatric healthcare landscape, there will be more rigour around these technologies and they will continue to be evaluated for their effectiveness in clinical practice and impact on patient outcomes
- The field is wide open, with many exciting tech projects on the horizon making the healthcare future more exciting. Undoubtedly, there is a great need for clinicians to be closely involved in developing solutions which are patient focussed and user friendly. The future is digital and has only just begun.

# REFERENCES

1.  Zimlichman E, Nicklin W, Aggarwal R, Bates DW. Health care 2030: The coming transformation. NEJM Catal: Innovat Care Delivery 2021.
2.  Bates DW, Singh H. Two decades since To Err Is Human: an assessment of progress and emerging priorities in patient safety. Health Aff (Millwood) 2018; 37:1736–1743.
3.  HM Government. Genome UK: the future of healthcare. 2020. https://assets.publishing.service. gov.uk/government/uploads/system/uploads/attachment_data/file/920378/Genome_UK_-_the_ future_of_healthcare.pdf (Last accessed 18th January 2023).
4.  NHS. Topol review. 2017. https://www.hee.nhs.uk/our-work/topol-review (Last accessed 18th January 2023).
5.  Wong BLH, Khurana MP, Smith RD, et al. Harnessing the digital potential of the next generation of health professionals. Hum Resour Health 2021; 19:50.
6.  Dang A, Arora D, Rane P. Role of digital therapeutics and the changing future of healthcare. J Family Med Prim Care 2020; 9:2207–13.
7.  https://www.dimesociety.org/about-us/Defining Digital Medicine/
8.  Digital Therapeutics Alliance. Understanding Dtx: What is a DTx. 2022. https://dtxalliance.org/ understanding-dtx/what-is-a-dtx/ (Last accessed 18th January 2023).
9.  DigitalHealth London. Digital Therapeutics in the NHS: The rise of digital therapies and the evidence that proves they work. https://digitalhealth.london/wp-content/uploads/2018/04/ DigitalTherapeuticsNHS.pdf (Last accessed 18th January 2023).
10. GOV.UK. Guidance: In vitro diagnostic medical devices: guidance on legislation. https://www.gov. uk/government/publications/in-vitro-diagnostic-medical-devices-guidance-on-legislation. (Last accessed 18th January 2023).
11. https://eumdr.com/guidance/ The European Union Medical Device Regulation Regulation (EU) 2017/745 (EU MDR)

12. US Food and Drug Administration. International Medical Device Regulators Forum (IMDRF). 2019. https://www.fda.gov/medical-devices/cdrh-international-programs/international-medical-device-regulators-forum-imdrf (last accessed 18th January 2023).

13. Benson T, Grieve G. Principles of health interoperability: SNOMED CT, HL7 and FHIR. Germany: Springer, 2016.

14. NHS 75 Digital. Digital child health implementation guides. 2021. https://digital.nhs.uk/services/digital-child-health/digital-child-health implementation-guides/implementing-child-health-interoperability-step-by-step-guide (Last accessed 18th January 2023).

15. Science Daily. No wires, more cuddles: Sensors are first to monitor babies in the NICU without wires. 2019. https://www.sciencedaily.com/releases/2019/02/190228141243.htm (Last accessed 18th January 2023).

16. Choudhary R. Sepsis Management, Controversies, and Advancement in Nanotechnology: A Systematic Review. Cureus 2022; 14:e22112.

17. Russo E, Spallarossa A, Tasso B, Villa C, Brullo C. Nanotechnology for Pediatric Retinoblastoma Therapy. Pharmaceuticals 2022; 15:1087.

18. Kouroupa A, Laws KR, Irvine K, et al. The use of social robots with children and young people on the autism spectrum: A systematic review and meta-analysis. PLoS One 2022; 17:e0269800.

19. Stern AD, Brönneke J, Debatin JF, et al. Advancing digital health applications: priorities for innovation in real-world evidence generation. The Lancet 2022; 4:E200–E206.

20. Vijayavenkataraman S, Fuh JYH, Lu WF. 3D Printing and 3D Bioprinting in Pediatrics. Bioengineering (Basel) 2017; 4:63.

21. Hazlett H, Gu H, Munsell B, et al. Early brain development in infants at high risk for autism spectrum disorder. Nature 2017; 542:348–351.

22. World Health Organizations. Global strategy on digital health 2020–2025. 2021. https://www.who.int/docs/default source/documents/gs4dhdaa2a9f352b0445bafbc79ca799dce4d.pdf (Last accessed 18th January 2023).

23. Kickbusch I, Piselli D, Agrawal A, et al. The Lancet and Financial Times Commission on governing health futures 2030: growing up in a digital world. The Lancet. 2021; 398:P1727–1776.

24. Peppin A, Thomas C. Health datafication, digital phenotyping and the 'Internet of Health': A new report from the Ada Lovelace Institute explores the datafication of health, how it manifests and the consequences for people and society. https://www.adalovelaceinstitute.org/blog/health-datafication-digital-phenotyping-and-the-internet-of-health/ (Last accessed 18th January 2023).

25. Ramgopal S, Sanchez-Pinto LN, Horvat CM, et al. Artificial intelligence-based clinical decision support in pediatrics. Pediatr Res 2022.

26. Hoffman HG , Seibel EJ, Richards TL, et al. Virtual reality helmet display quality influences the magnitude of virtual reality analgesia. J Pain 2006; 7:843–850.

27. Hoffman HG, Doctor JN, Patterson DR, Carrougher GJ, Furness TA 3rd. Virtual reality as an adjunctive pain control during burn wound care in adolescent patients. Pain 2000; 85:305–309.

28. Shepherd K, Shanmugharaj Y, Kattan O, Kokkinakis M. Can virtual reality headsets be used safely as a distraction method for paediatric orthopaedic patients? A feasibility study. Ann R Coll Surg Engl 2022; 104:144–147.

29. The 4 Phases of Double Diamond approach https://www.designcouncil.org.uk/our-work/skills-learning/the-double-diamond/

30. Sushmitha S, Tanushree Devi B, Mahesh V, et al. Virtual reality therapy in prolonging attention spans for ADHD. Advan Biomed Engineer Technol 2021:391–400.